The Illustrated Compendium of

Prosthetic Heart Valves

The Illustrated Compendium of

Prosthetic Heart Valves

AMIT BANERJEE
Professor of Cardiovascular-thoracic Surgery
Govind Ballabh Pant Hospital
Maulana Azad Medical College
UNIVERSITY OF DELHI

Academic Foundation
NEW DELHI

Disclaimer : The illustrations used in this publication have been principally acquired from the following categories of sources: previous publications such as periodicals (newsletters, newspapers, magazines, journals); and books (textbooks, reference volumes) either copyrighted or in the public domain; declared, assumed or apparent public domain sites on the World Wide Web; manufacturers'/vendors' websites; physicians'/surgeons' websites; institutional websites; educational websites; device catalogues and pamphlets issued by manufacturers/vendors; personally requisitioned from individual physicians/ surgeons/scientists/curators/collectors/others on condition of appropriate acknowledgment or on condition of anonymity; abandoned/unclaimed scrap. Adequate care has been taken to obtain permission for publication of copyrighted material in book as well as electronic format in a CD-Rom. Each such permission has been duly acknowledged by the author in the book and the accompanying CD-Rom. However, the likely possibility of copyrighted images having inadvertently crept in through other sources cannot be denied. Whenever any such instance of unintentional copyright infringement is brought to the author or publisher's attention, appropriate and immediate corrective action feasible under the circumstances is assured. Since this publication and the accompanying CD-Rom are chiefly intended to be instruments for educational activities, they are eminently protected within limitations on exclusive rights, as detailed in the 'Fair use statute' of prevalent copyright norms.

All information presented in the publication is obtained from sources believed by the author to be accurate and reliable. Although reasonable care has been taken to ensure that the information herein is true, such information is provided 'as is', without any warranty express or implied as to the accuracy, timeliness or completeness of any such information. Neither the publisher nor the author shall be liable for any losses incurred by users from any use of this publication or its contents.

First Published in 2004 by

ACADEMIC FOUNDATION

4772-73 / 23 Bharat Ram Road
(23 Ansari Road), Darya Ganj
New Delhi - 110 002
INDIA

Phones : +91-11-23245001, 02, 03, 04.
Fax : +91-11-23245005
e-mail : academic@vsnl.com
www : academicfoundation.com

The Illustrated Compendium of Prosthetic Heart Valves
Amit Banerjee
ISBN 81-7188-334-6
(Book + CD-Rom)

Designed and typeset by Academic Foundation
Printed and bound at Print Perfect, New Delhi

I dedicate this book to

My peers

To those who bucked me up at every stage

And even more

To those who derided my efforts as futile

Contents

Foreword

Soon after extracorporeal circulation first allowed unhurried surgery on the open heart, surgeons and engineers began to chase a dream of making artificial heart valves that would do the job that nature does so well. It never was simply a matter of a mechanism that allowed fluid to flow in one direction only. The many subtle and not so subtle interactions between the blood and the materials used to make valves, the healing of the host to the device, the rheology of blood flow through the valve and the dynamic effects on the moving parts of valves and vice versa, the microscopic but considerable forces generated by the opening and closing of some devices, all have contributed to the failure to reach the holy grail of a replacement device that truly did everything that the natural valve does.

Dr Amit Banerjee has taken on the task of chronicling these efforts. It is a monumental task but a most worthy one. The range of ingenuity sometimes imitating nature and sometimes ignoring her that has been displayed in the design of the mechanisms, and the endless search for materials that will match and survive the conditions of the human body, are all on display. This book will serve as a memorial to the creativity and perseverance of those who have tried and failed to find the perfect valve and yet who by their efforts have prolonged the lives of so many victims of heart valve disease. It can be an inspiration to those who will in the future finally reach that goal. The difficulties facing Dr Banerjee have been enormous. Only by great persistence and the expenditure of much energy could this task have been completed. We owe him our congratulations and our gratitude for an important job well done.

It is novel and laudable that the publication has a companion CD-Rom to show many of the valves in their true colours; there will also be periodic updates through the publisher's website. Let us hope that the results of the author's enthusiasm, energy and dogged persistence will be found useful by budding cardiac surgeons.

Bronx, NY, USA ROBERT WILLIAM MAYO FRATER *MS FRCS*

Preface

Half a century has elapsed since Charles Hufnagel's historic feat of inserting a ball valve device into the descending thoracic aorta of a patient with severe aortic regurgitation. Applauding this monumental accomplishment, Edward A Lefrak and Albert Starr, in their book *Cardiac Valve Prostheses*, wrote, "Hufnagel ignited the fire of prosthetic valve implantation...". No less creditable however were the relentless efforts and perseverance of his peers and successors, many of whom remained unsung.

Nearly fifty years have also passed since Dwight Emary Harken enumerated his 'Ten Commandments' for the ideal prosthetic heart valve. It is ironic, and indicative of the limitations of man and his science, that these criteria continue to be universally quoted but still remain unfulfilled. Incredible strides like robotics, port access and genetic engineering notwithstanding, a heart valve prosthesis which is "safer than the condition it corrects", remains a mirage. Yet, the failures fail to frustrate; the spirit refuses to die; enthusiasm scents triumph at the very next step... as efforts continue unabated.

> "We shall not cease from exploration
> And the end of all our exploring
> Will be to arrive where we started
> And know the place for the first time"

Eliot's lines are particularly applicable to this ongoing evolution of heart valve prostheses.

The publication in your hands is a humble attempt to place on record the outcome of these efforts. There is no value judgment here; no quantification of failures or successes. Indeed, each failure has only represented success in eliminating a possible future failure; and every success has only served as a reminder that perfection is yet to materialise. How far the efforts expended between the covers of this book have succeeded will be measured by the number of readers who write in to point out its lapses. In order to keep the doors wide open for such communication, a companion CD-Rom is provided. Once registered, the reader can enjoy on-line updates on the subject and fresh inputs can be shared.

It is singularly fortunate that another legend of our times, who has devoted almost fifty years of incessant efforts towards the amelioration of heart valve disease, has lent his pen for the Foreword of this book. No author could ever hope for one with better credentials for the job than Professor RWM Frater.

It needs to be emphasised that in bringing out this book, I have played the role of a mere facilitator. The credit goes to all those authors, webmasters and correspondents whose assets have lent strength to its foundation.

New Delhi, India — Amit Banerjee *MS MCh*

The Trailblazers

"Surgery of the heart has probably reached the limit set by nature to all surgery; no new method and no new discovery can overcome the natural difficulties that attend a wound of the heart." Thus foretold Dr Christian Billroth in Dr Stephen Paget's textbook *Surgery of the Chest*. Defying his prophecy, Dr Ludwig Rehn of Frankfurt, Germany, succeeded in sewing up a right ventricular stab wound in in a 22–year–old man in September, 1896. As the French duo of Drs Eugene Doyen and Marin Théodore Tuffier, and Harvard surgeon Dr Elliott Cutler, ventured to tackle stenotic pulmonary (1913), aortic (1914) and mitral (1923) valves respectively, the formidable bastion of valvular heart disease suffered the first chinks in its masonry. The next two–and–a–half decades saw human enterprise overcome many a congenital and acquired cardiovascular condition; yet, the quandary of managing patients with severely diseased, repair–defying cardiac valves kept haunting clinicians ....till began the fascinating saga of prosthetic heart valves.

The pre–extracorporeal era

The endeavour of fabricating a surrogate device to replace an irreparably diseased natural heart valve began in right earnest after the Second World War. Dr Charles A Hufnagel[1] of Georgetown University Medical Center, Washington, DC started his experiments with a ball–valve device in 1946. Subsequently he ushered in the era of human artificial heart valve implantation on 11 September, 1952 by inserting a methyl methacrylate (commercially available as Lucite/Perspex/Plexiglass) tube and ball device *(Figure 001)* in the descending thoracic aorta of a patient with severe aortic regurgitation. This was before extracorporeal technology was applied on human subjects. In principle, his device resembled a bottle stopper *(Figure 002)* for which a patent was obtained by JB Williams[2] in 1858. Hufnagel's valve was held in place by specially designed fixation rings which facilitated rapid insertion of the device with minimal duration of aortic clamping. These rings utilised the principle of 'multiple point fixation' to avoid necrosis of the aortic wall. Around the same time, Dr J Moore Campbell[3] of Oklahoma City had independently experimented with a similar device *(Figure 003)* in dogs. Why he never employed his valve in man is not clear. Hufnagel had also experimented awhile, albeit on a discouraging note, with homologous aortic valve grafts; but Dr Conrad C Lam[4] and compatriots from the Henry Ford Hospital, Detroit, Michigan reported success with this

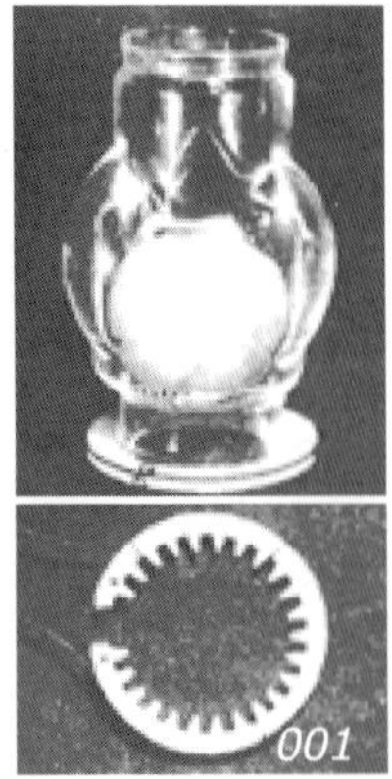

001

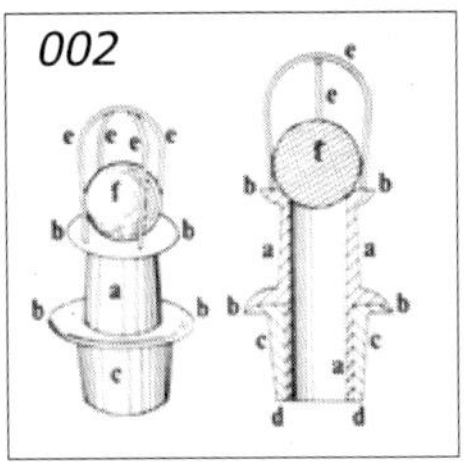

002

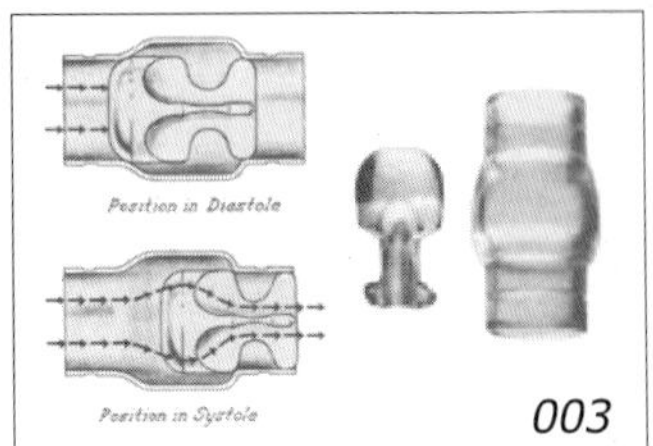

003

004

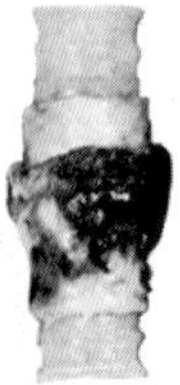

technique in 74 dogs. They had ingeniously sutured a short cuff of aorta to the myocardial end of the harvested canine aortic valve. Prior to its insertion into the descending aorta, a grooved Lucite or polythene tube was attached at either end *(Figure 004)*. Dr Gordon Murray[5] of the Toronto General Hospital experimented with the direct insertion of canine aortic valve segments into the descending aorta *(Figure 005).* Later he became the first to carry out such a procedure in a human subject. He obtained the homograft from the cadaver of a 32–year–old man, and implanted into the descending aorta of a 22–year–old man in October 1955. Meanwhile Dr Norman E Shumway's group[6] at the Stanford University School of Medicine, Palo Alto, California had begun their experiments with pulmonary valve autotransplantation which included using it as a mitral valve substitute.[7] Hufnagel's device continued to be inserted till 1958. He changed the material of the ball to silicone rubber moulded over a hollow nylon core. This lowered the noise level, and the reduced weight of the ball made it more sensitive to pressure changes. For patients in whom clamping of the descending aorta was undesirable, Dacron (wrinkle–resistant synthetic polyester) or Teflon (polytetrafluoroethylene–PTFE) tubing sleeves were added to facilitate placement of the device as a permanent bypass *(Figure 006)*.

005

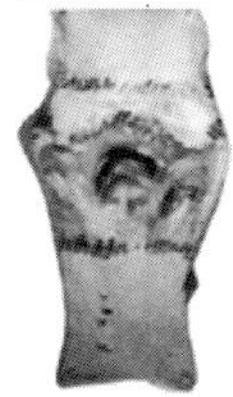

The problem of mitral regurgitation also received zealous attention from several quarters. In 1950, Dr G Rehmi Denton[8] of the Albany Medical

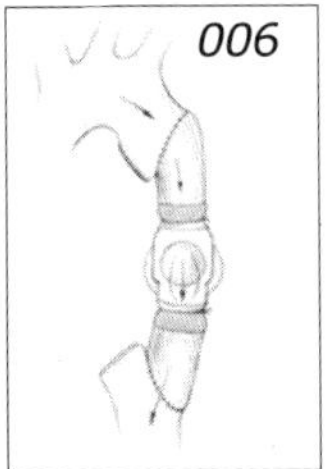

006

college, New York designed three types *(Figure 007)* of polyethylene plastic mitral valve prostheses for his canine experiments. These one-piece devices aimed at containment of regurgitation, by the ventricular wall partially occluding a central tubular flow channel during systole. Dr Dwight Emary Harken[9] of the Peter Bent Brigham Hospital, Boston, Massachussetts tried placing intraventricular Lucite spheres beneath the posterior mitral leaflet in the hope of limiting the severity of regurgitation. He also inserted spindle–shaped baffles in the mitral orifice to compensate for loss of valve tissue. It was Harken[10] who had the vision to spell out the 'Ten Commandments' on what should, in the long run, constitute an 'ideal' heart valve prosthesis. On 22 July, 1955, Dr Judson T Chesterman performed the first human mitral valve implantation at the City General Hospital in Sheffield, England.[11] It was a closed–heart procedure. The device *(Figure 008)* was made of Perspex, and consisted of an outer cage and a poppet. Two buttons attached to the prosthesis allowed it to be fastened to the outside of the heart. The patient lived for 14 hours after the operation, but died when the poppet got twisted out of position. Another pioneering effort was that of Murray,[5] who reportedly used a closed heart method of implanting an aortic valve homograft in the mitral position in a human subject, after initial canine experiments *(Figure 009)*.

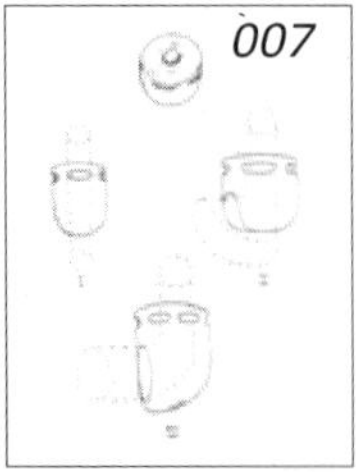

007

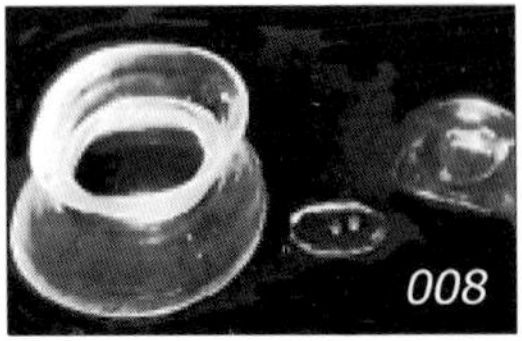

008

Enter the heart–lung machine

009

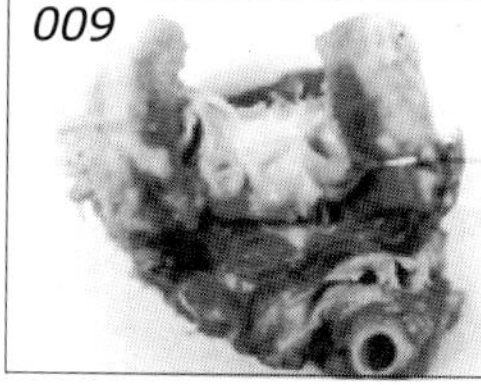

The first known human open heart operation involving an artificial heart–lung device was performed by Dr Clarence Dennis at the University of Minnesota Medical School, Minneapolis, Minnesota in 1951. In 1952, Dr John Lewis[12] from the same centre initiated open heart surgery under hypothermia and inflow occlusion. In the same year, Dr Forest D Dodrill, a surgeon at the Wayne State University's Harper Hospital in Detroit, used extracorporeal equipment designed by General Motors on a patient. In 1953, Dr C Walton Lillehei, also of the University of Minnesota Medical School, was the first to use controlled cross-circulatory support for open heart surgery while Dr John Gibbon, Jr of the Jefferson Medical College Hospital, Philadelphia, Pennsylvania successfully repaired an atrial septal defect with the help of a heart–lung machine. The first direct valve repair operation under cardiopulmonary bypass is credited to Lillehei.[13]

Quest for an aortic valve replacement device

Although it took quite a few years for cardiopulmonary bypass to attain wide application, it paved the way for further research on valvular prostheses. Hufnagel[14] experimented with ways to modify his device to make it suitable for insertion at the aortic valvar level. He added multiple fenestrations (to facilitate coronary perfusion) to his ball–valve device and secured it with a tape tied around the base of the aorta, proximal to

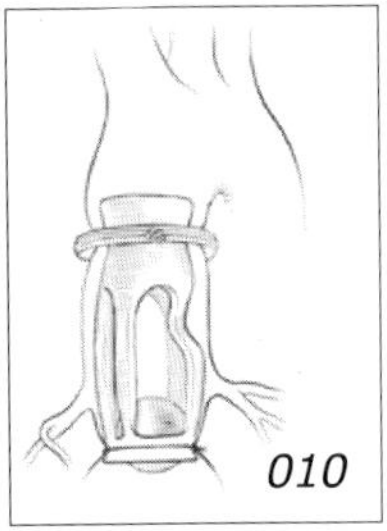

010

the coronary ostia *(Figure 010)*. This experimental prototype was further modified by replacing the ball occluder with a helical coil spring *(Figure 011)*, to improve haemodynamic performance. Another group, led by Dr W Sterling Edwards[15] of the Medical College of Alabama, Birmingham, was also engaged in canine experiments with a subcoronary ball–valve prosthesis *(Figure 012)*.

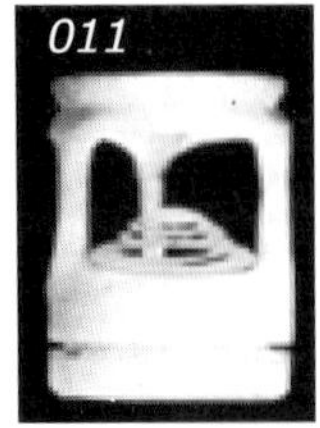

011

Many of the initial efforts to develop an orthotopic prosthetic heart valve aimed at mimicking the mechanical characteristics of a natural heart valve. Flexible polyurethanes and silicone rubber materials were popular on account of their easy availability and handling. In 1953, Mr David Moore of the Research and Development Laboratory at the University of California, San Francisco, developed precision–tooled moulds for pressure injection of various extrudable materials. A General Electric elastomer was selected for fabrication of a cylinder–mounted three-cusp valve *(Figure 013)*. In 1954, Dr Benson B Roe[16] from the same university started animal experiments with this device, which was inserted through a descending aortotomy and then manipulated into the ascending aorta where it was fixed with sutures. Around 1955,

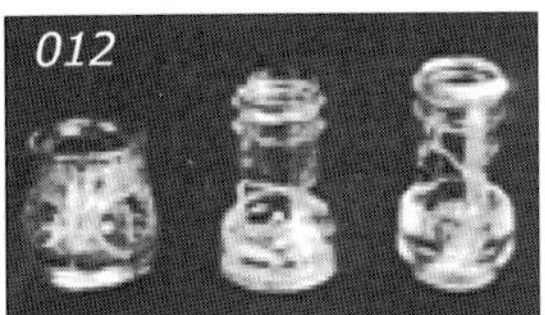

012

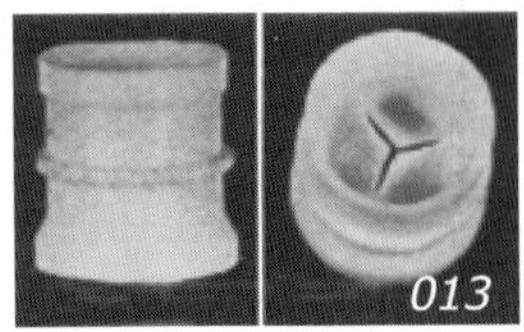

013

Hufnagel started working on a trileaflet replica *(Figure 014)* of the aortic valve fabricated out of various materials including silicone rubber and silicone-on-Dacron mesh. The three cusps were held together by a central ring which was anchored to the aortic wall at a suitable distance from the valve. This particular model had a couple of human successes. Drs Earle B Kay and Akio Suzuki of St Vincent Charity Hospital, Cleveland, Ohio put in serious efforts towards the development of prosthetic heart valves. In the process they tried out three designs of aortic valve prostheses of which the first was developed in 1957.[17] It had coronary side arms *(Figure 015)* built into the artificial valve that provided for coronary artery transposition above the valve leaflets. Cuffs of aortic wall were excised around the coronary ostia to which the artificial coronary arteries were anastomosed. The artificial valve was then sutured to the proximal and distal cuffs of the aorta.

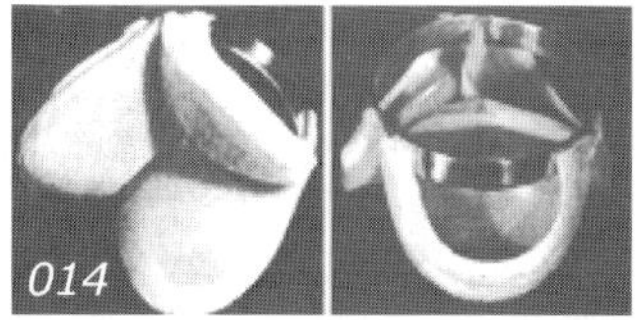

014

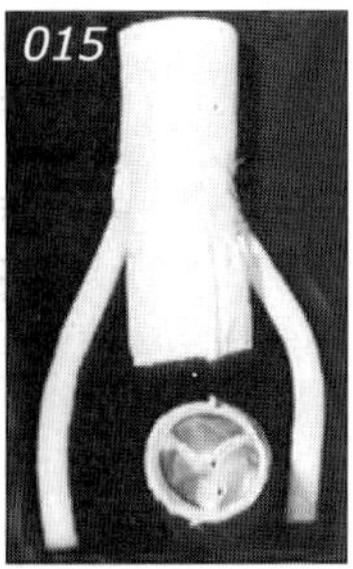

015

The next design to be used in the subcoronary position consisted of three triangular leaflets with a semicircular base for attachment *(Figure 016)*. The fabric used was porous knitted Teflon lightly filmed with a solution of 15% polyurethane, dissolved in tetrahydrofuran. The resultant material was smooth and nonporous. A 4 mm margin,

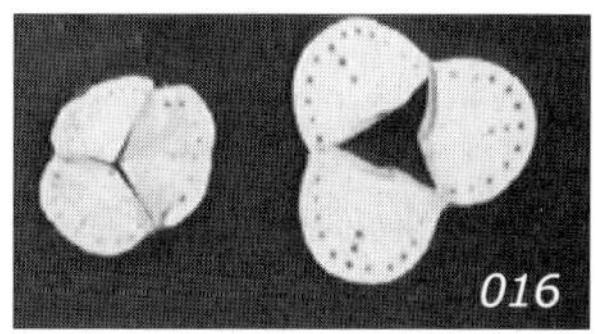

016

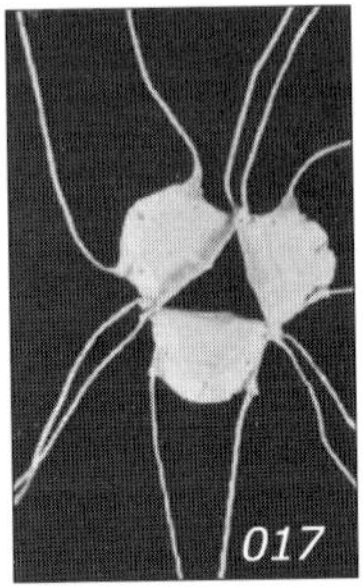

017

free of polyurethane, was maintained at the edge of the leaflets to provide porosity for tissue ingrowth which would lead to permanency of tissue fixation. The third design was a modification of the second. The leaflet fabric had 5 mm wide extensions which tapered to cords about 15 cm long and 1 mm wide *(Figure 017).* These cords were threaded and passed through the aortic wall and tied with the corresponding one from the adjacent leaflet over pledgets of Teflon felt. All three designs were used on human subjects with mixed results. Meanwhile, Dr Henry T Bahnson[18] of the Johns Hopkins University Hospital, Baltimore, Maryland, Roe[19] and others obtained encouraging experimental results with individual cusp substitutes made out of scalloped Teflon *(Figure 018),* compression moulded Silastic (silicone rubber), and other materials. Harken tried similar cusp substitutes made out of Teflon and polyurethane but was not satisfied. A flexible trileaflet silicone–rubber and mesh prosthesis *(Figure 019)* designed by Roe was used for a limited clinical trial from 1960 onwards.[20] It had a Dacron tape sewing ring. Dr JC van der Spuy[21] from the University of Pretoria, South Africa designed a clamp *(Figure 020)* and devised a formula to harvest autogenous

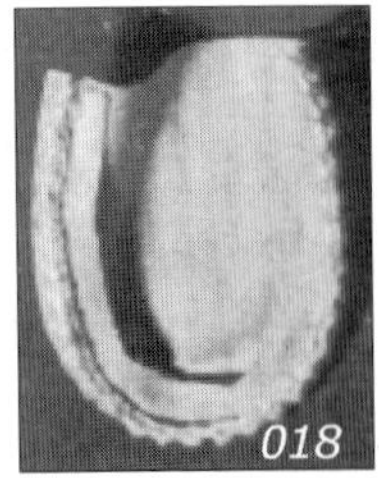

018

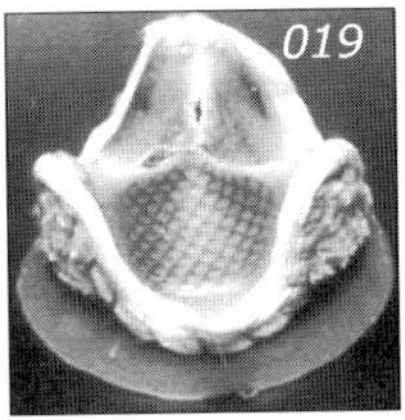

019

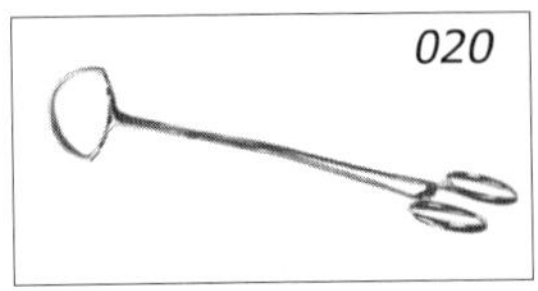

020

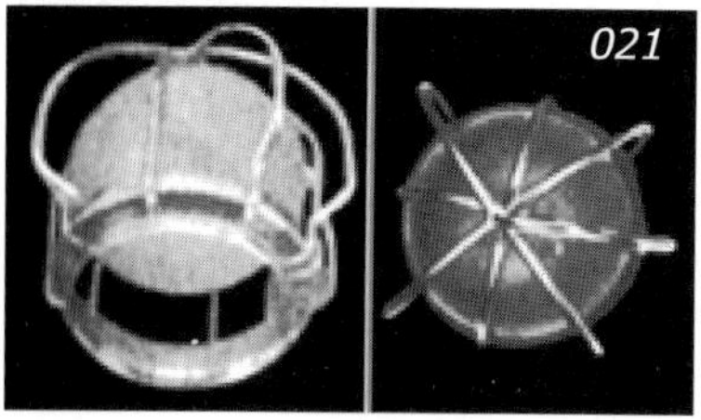

pericardial cusps to repair the aortic valve.

On 10 March, 1960, Harken implanted a 'ball and double cage' aortic valve prosthesis *(Figure 021)* in the subcoronary position in a patient with severe aortic insufficiency.[22] The outer cage aimed at allaying any possibility of poppet movement interference by the aortic wall. The stainless steel cage initially enclosed a Lucite ball which was later changed to silicone-rubber. The device was anchored with Surgaloy and a sewing ring created with Ivalon or Teflon backing. About half a dozen of these valves were implanted in quick succession. Later, he tried out modified versions of his ball valve.[23] Human implantation of Roe and Moore's elastomer valve was performed in the subcoronary position under cardiopulmonary bypass in July, 1960.[16]

Drs Dwight C McGoon and Emerson A Moffitt[24] from the Mayo Clinic, Rochester, Minnesota carried out total reconstruction of the aortic valve with the help of a round tube knitted from 200–denier Teflon strands. A trileaflet prosthesis fashioned from this tube *(Figure 022)* was fixed to the native aortic annulus with the help of about 15 interrupted mattress sutures of 3–0 silk in each cusp.

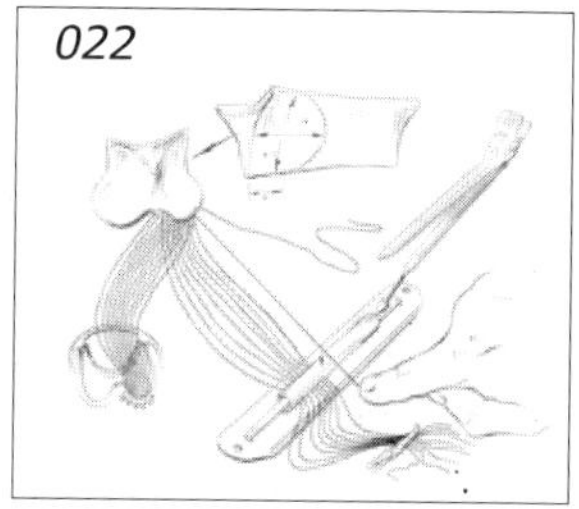

Crusade for a suitable atrioventricular valve substitute

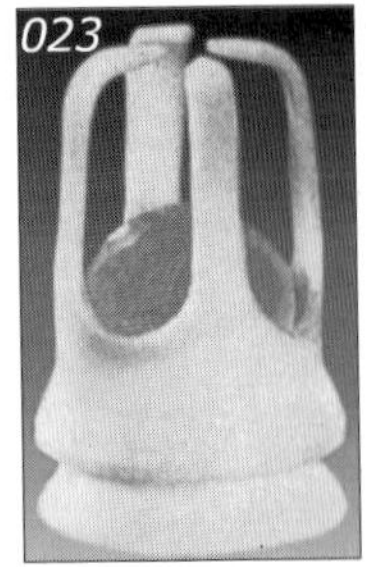

023

Dr MC Kernan (working with Dennis, now at the University of New York College of Medicine) and colleagues[25] fabricated a mitral valve comprising a Lucite ball in a Teflon cage *(Figure 023)*, which was implanted in 25 dogs on a fibrillating heart under cardiopulmonary bypass. Drs F Henry Ellis, Jr and AH Bulbulian[26] of the Mayo Clinic had designed a Perspex caged ball prosthesis *(Figure 024)* and also a Teflon pivoted disc *(Figure 025)* prosthesis, both used only for canine experiments.[27] A similar all Teflon device *(Figure 026)* had also been designed by Dr Bruce C Paton from the University of Colorado Medical Center, Denver. In 1958, Dr Louis Schwab[28] of the University of Cincinnati College of Medicine, Cincinnati, Ohio reportedly fabricated a ball valve for experimental use *(Figure 027)*, constructed totally out of highly compressed Ivalon mounted on a stainless steel frame. The ball had a stainless steel pin to serve as a radio-opaque marker. Dr EH Berg and colleagues from the State University of New York College of Medicine reported the experimental use of a

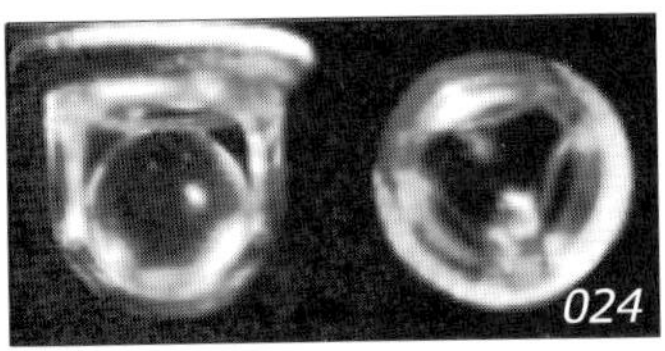

024

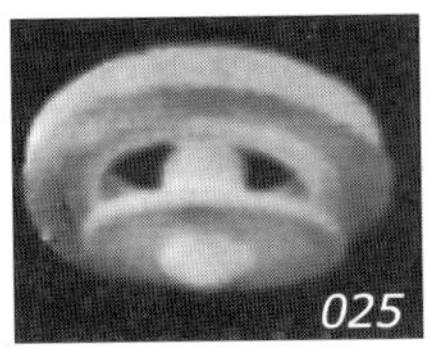

025

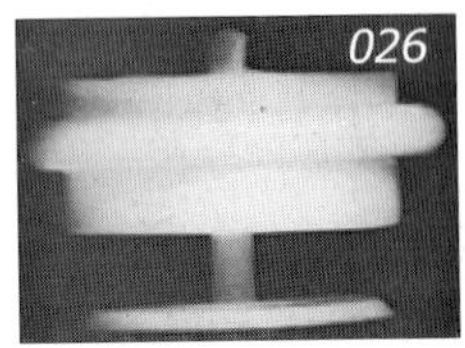

026

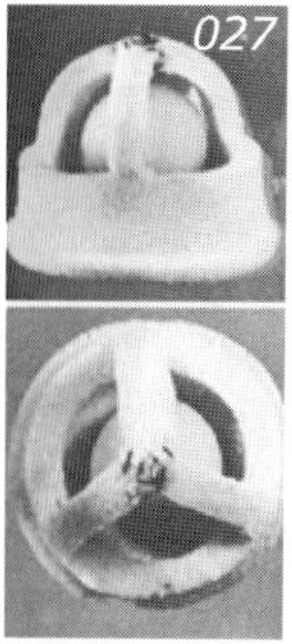
027

flap-valve prosthesis *(Figure 028)*, fabricated from a combination of metal and plastic, to replace the mitral valve. At the Mayo Clinic, Rochester, Minnesota, Dr Robert WM Frater,[29 30] along with Ellis, began developing a flexible monocusp valve in 1959. Initially, the material used was silicone rubber. It had a D-shaped ring; the straight portion was aligned with the base of the excised anterior cusp. The artificial cusp was attached to the straight side of the ring and had hinges parallel to this. Between the hinges, the rigid portions of the cusp met the ventricular surface of the ring in closing. Subsequently the valve was made of layers of laminated Mylar and joined by Schjelbond glue. It had central flow and was, with its flexible cusp, a hybrid polymer/mechanical device *(Figure 029)*. Ellis and Dr Ara V Doumanian,[31] a research fellow, also experimented with a coating of open-cell polyurethane foam to cover the surfaces of this prosthesis. At the Cleveland Clinic Foundation, Drs Tetsuzo Akutsu and Barend Dreyer from Dr Willem J Kolff's group experimented with polyurethane[32] and Teflon fabric siliconised with Siliclad.[33] They used tricuspid semilunar valve moulds to fabricate the device which was mounted on a stainless steel screen ring covered with polyurethane sponge *(Figure 030)*. Dr Christiaan N Barnard of the Groote Schuur Hospital, University

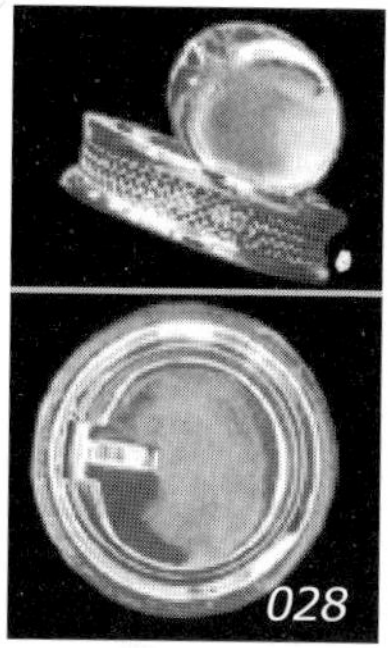
028

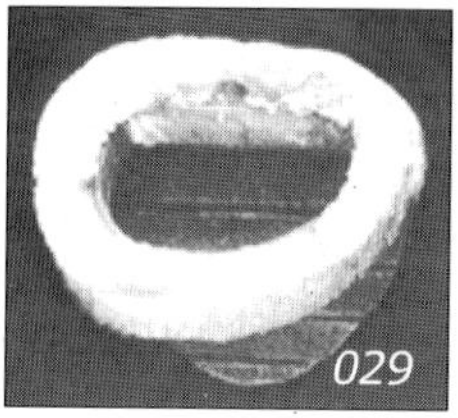
029

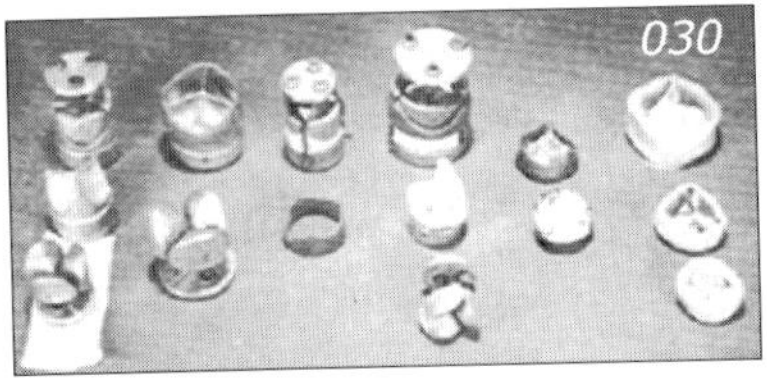

030

of Cape Town, tried a Silastic flap device *(Figure 031)* to replace the posterior mitral leaflet in dogs.[34] van der Spuy tried reconstructing the mitral valve as well from autogenous tissues.[35] For this purpose he developed a clamp–cutter device

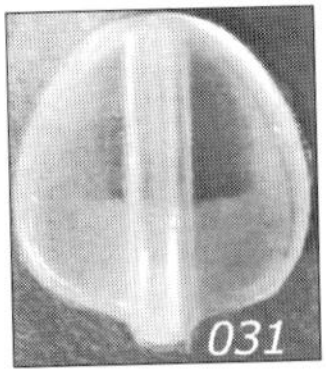

031

(Figure 032) to tailor a valve out of autologous pericardium, attached to two sets of chordae tendineae—meticulously fashioned out of the iliotibial tract *(Figure 033)*. Replacement of individual mitral valve leaflets with either autogenous pericardium or synthetic material such as Ivalon also received active consideration.[36,37,38,39]

In all probability, the first human mitral valve replacement under cardiopulmonary bypass[40] was performed by Dr Nina S Braunwald at the National Heart Institute, Bethesda, Maryland on 11 March 1960, one day after Harken's first aortic ball valve implant. Dr. Stephen Westaby,[41]

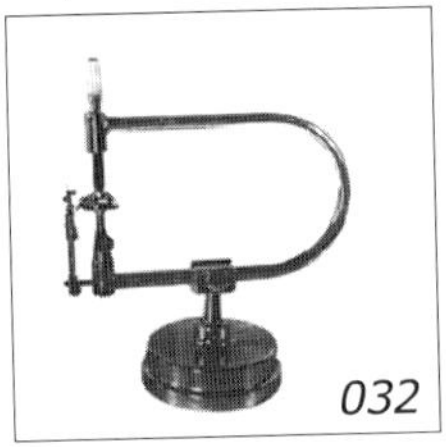

032

in his book *Landmarks in Cardiac Surgery* mentions this date also as 10 March 1960. She used a polyurethane valve reinforced with Dacron *(Figure 034)*. Using a plastic steel

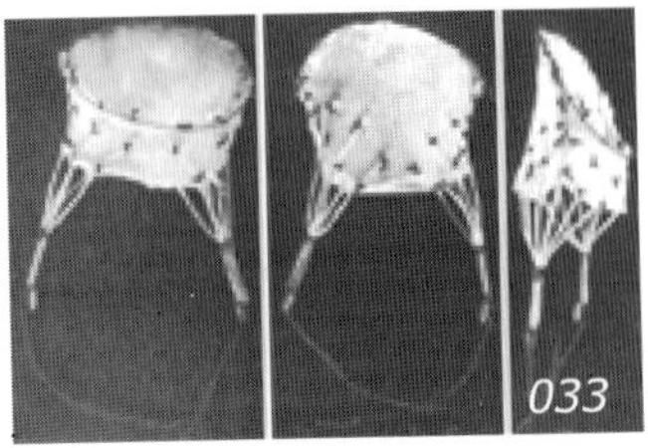

033

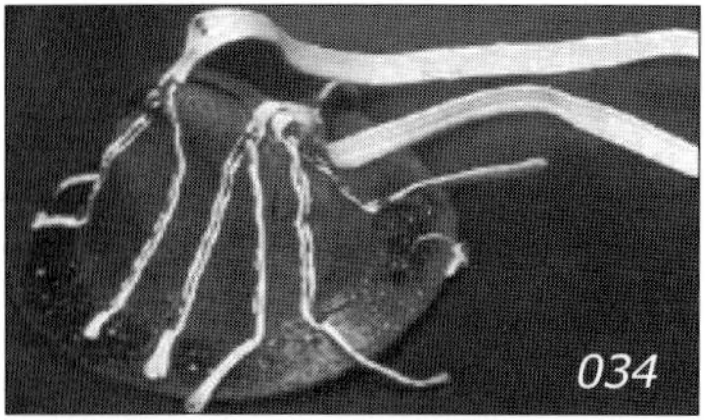
034

called Devcon, two-piece moulds from which the finished valves were to be fabricated were made. The valve had two leaflets. Teflon chordae attached to the device were brought out through the ventricular muscle and secured outside the heart at the time of implantation. Frater's flexible monocusp underwent first human implantation on 16 July 1960. To encourage neointima formation, which would reduce the chances of thromboembolism, the device was covered with knitted Dacron fabric. Historically, this was the first low-profile, fabric-covered valve. Dr Viking Olov Björk of the Karolinska Institute, Stockholm, Sweden, lauded it as the very first application of the principle of tilting disc valves.[42]

The cornerstone had been laid, and the quest for a sure-fire prosthetic valve had gathered abundant momentum. Blueprints were essayed and new materials investigated. Breakthroughs pepped, but the frustrations hardly ever failed to provoke renewed efforts. During the sixties, a number of innovative designs were pieced together for experimental as well as clinical application.

The Stokers

The flame ignited by the pioneers did exactly what the sacred waters of Fount Hippocrence do to poets; it kindled the sprits of creation, innovation and motivation to weave and forge spare parts for the heart. Medical scientists and biomedical engineers — independently and collectively — stoked, and the tinder obliged.

Bileaflet valves

In 1958, Dr John Holter (an honorary DSc having been conferred on him), an engineer by profession, who had invented the Spitz–Holter valve for hydrocephalus, had drawn the sketch of a bileaflet silicone heart valve in his notebook *(Figure 035)*. Presumably, the idea occurred to him for possible future application in the silicone artificial heart, fabricated in collaboration with Dr Frank Hastings. There is no evidence to suggest that the concept ever graduated to a prototype. Around the same time, Dr Albert Starr of the University of Oregon, Portland and Miles Lowell Edwards, a retired engineer, whose ultimate goal was an implantable artificial heart, teamed up to chase the dream of an ideal heart valve substitute. Their maiden venture was a bileaflet valve which consisted of two silicone–rubber leaflets hinged on a central cross-bar made of solid Teflon *(Figure 036)*; it included a Teflon cloth margin for fixation. Animal experiments with this model were plagued by thrombus formation.

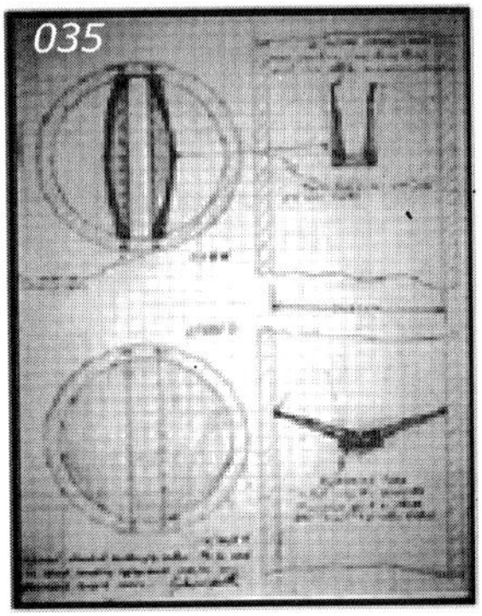

Frustrated, Starr and Edwards abandoned the project.[43]

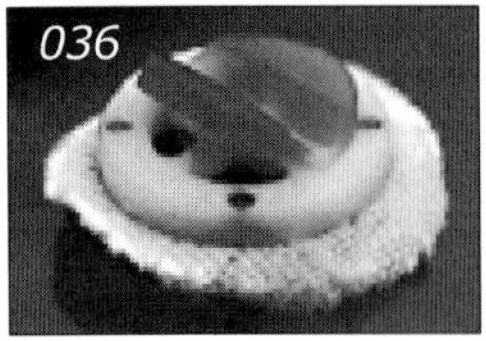

In the early sixties, Dr Vincent Gott of the University of Wisconsin, Madison and Ronald L Daggett, an engineer, designed a new bileaflet valve. The device had a Lexan (polycarbonate) housing and centrally hinged, flexible 'butterfly wing' leaflets anchored to a cross strut *(Figure 037)*. The leaflets were fabricated from a 'wafer' of Teflon fabric with an additional laminate of percale applied to their non-hinging area. The fabric in the leaflet was Silastic-impregnated. Lateral stabilisation was ensured by two small stainless steel pins placed through the leaflet. A graphite-benzalkonium-heparin coating was applied to the housing of the valve. The first human implantation in the aortic position was done by Dr William P Young at the same institution on 30 April 1963. Unfortunately, the Gott-Daggett design was withdrawn from the market in 1965 after a few valves failed when the strut retaining the central flap came loose owing to assembly-related flaws.[44]

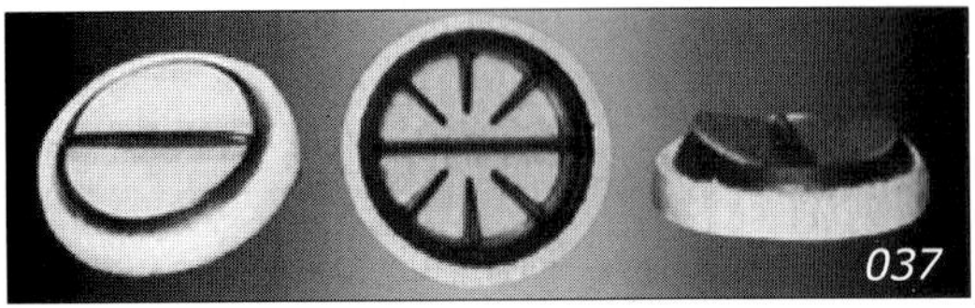

Gott further added to the cause of upcoming heart valves through his re-

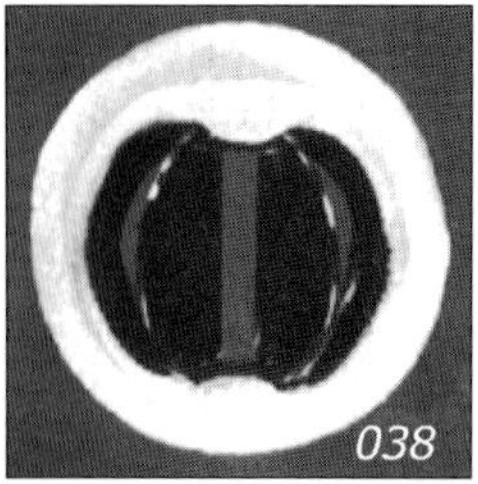

search in the field of thromboresistant biomaterials. His attempts to evaluate the biocompatibility of carbon led to the formation of a special division within a nuclear research company called General Atomics, charged with the mission of developing a durable form of carbon for use in implantable medical devices. In 1969, after more than six years of development, a new material called Pyrolite began to replace the plastic and metal materials that had been used for heart valve components.[45] Gott's contribution was of paramount importance because realisation was dawning that polymeric occluders suffered from degenerative failure. Silicone balls would absorb lipids from the blood stream and crack if not cured properly; Teflon was subject to failure through cold flow from repeated stress in a focussed location and Delrin (acetyl homopolymer) would warp in typical steam sterilisation cycles.[46]

Dr Bhagavant Kalke from India, while working with Dr C Walton Lillehei of the University of Minnesota Medical School, conceived the design of a low-profile bileaflet valve *(Figure 038)* in 1965. Initial prototypes of the device captured attention on account of superlative hydrodynamic performance in an analog pulse duplicator. This prosthesis had the leaflets opening to 60 degrees. As the leaflets opened they moved apart to create a central orifice, facilitating central laminar flow. Each leaflet had two short cylindrical cams that rotated within a semi–open ovoid recess in the orifice ring.[47] A few all–titanium models were handcrafted by Harry Cromie of Surgitool. One of these was used by Lillehei in the first and only clinical implantation in 1968. The patient died within 48 hours and the project was apparently put on the back burner.

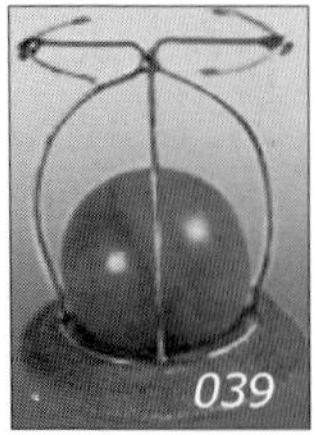

Ball and cage calves

Encouraged by the initial success of his double-caged aortic ball-valve, Harken tried out certain design modifications such as conversion to a single cage with two semicircular fences held in position by horizontal balusters *(Figure 039)*, ostensibly to prevent the ball from grazing the aortic wall; and later an open-caged model *(Figure 040)* suitable for both aortic and mitral positions.[22] The titanium cage had four tapered, ellipsoidal struts; the sewing ring was of four-ply Dacron and the Silastic ball was hollow.

The Oregon team designed an injection-moulded Lucite valve that had a multilaminated Teflon sewing ring attached with a stainless steel band. It had a solid Silastic ball. In the course of animal experiments, a snap-on Silastic shield *(Figure 041)*, which would cover the suture line and the injured endocardium on the atrial side, was given a try to reduce the incidence of thromboembolism.[48] The first human implantation of the Starr-Edwards ball and cage valve took place on 25 August 1960. The patient was a 33-year-old lady who had previously undergone a closed transventricular mitral commissurotomy and subsequent open

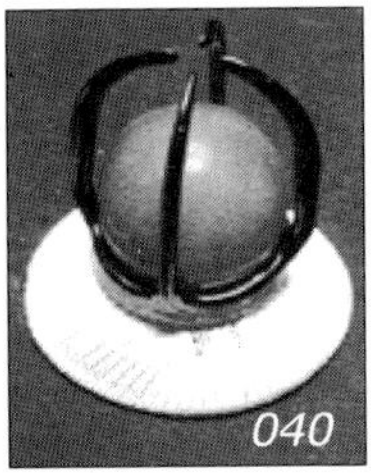

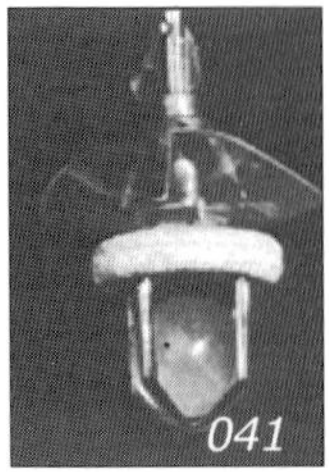

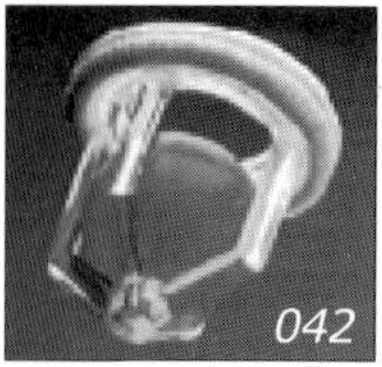

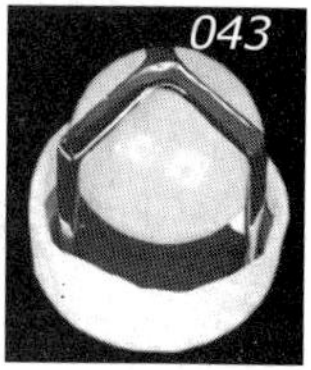

implantation of an Ivalon mitral leaflet. She had severe mitral regurgitation with pulmonary oedema. The operation was carried out through a right thoracotomy. The prosthesis used was modelled after the valve designed by Ellis and Bulbulian. It had a Lucite cage with thick struts and a machined ring orifice *(Figure 042)*. A compression-moulded silicone-rubber ball was placed inside the cage and the ring was then solvent-welded to the cage with acetone. The patient's immediate postoperative recovery was remarkable but 10 hours later she succumbed to massive air embolism, bringing into focus the very important issue of air trapped inside the heart after open heart surgery.[49] Starr and Edwards continued with their research and development in their quest for perfection. They also effected design modifications to make their valve suitable for aortic valve replacement. The Lucite cage gave way to stainless steel, which was subsequently replaced by an alloy called Stellite–21.[50] The initial prototypes *(Figure 043)* had relatively thin integrated sewing rings which were made bulkier, with an added Silastic ring in the later models

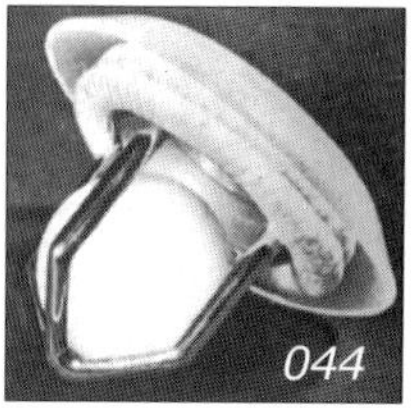

(Figure 044). With its encouraging clinical results, the Starr-Edwards valve was on its way to become the first commercially available prosthesis. Subsequent models of the valve, manufactured by the Edwards group, were numbered, starting with Model 1000 which had a Stellite–21 alloy single-cast cage with three metal 'feet' projecting into the centre of the orifice from the ring *(Figure 045)*. The closed apex cage had

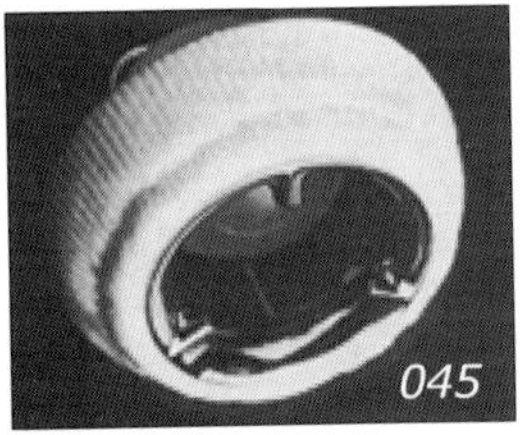

045

no welds, bends or hinges. The device had a Silastic ball and a Teflon sewing ring. Efforts to improve the valve's haemodynamic performance saw the introduction of Model 6000, which had no 'feet' but a

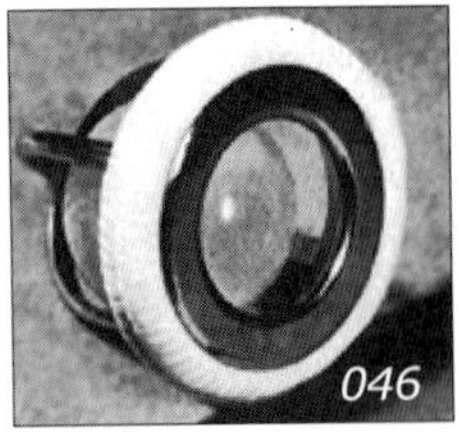

046

large ring of bare metal *(Figure 046)* at its orifice.[51] In 1966, Model 1260 aortic prosthesis *(Figure 047)* was introduced followed by its mitral counterpart (Model 6120) in 1968 *(Figure 048)*. The former had three struts in its cage while the latter had four. The sewing ring, made out of composite knitted Teflon and polypropylene cloth, was extended to the orifice, leaving no exposed metal on the inflow aspect of the valve. The struts were made thinner. The alloy cage was made from a single cast, so there were no welds, bends or hinges. The Silastic ball was impregnated with 2% barium sulphate for radio-opacity. Eventually this model was destined to establish its all-round superiority over the others. The year 1967 saw the introduction of Model 6300 with a totally Teflon fabric-covered cage and a polished electron-beam welded hollow ball made from Stellite *(Figure 049)*. The subsequent models incorporated

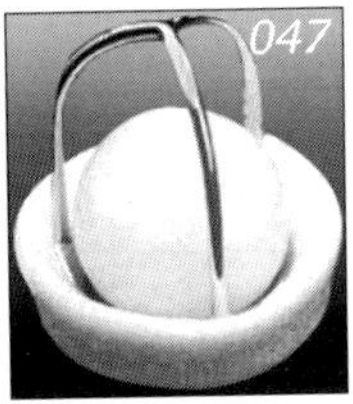

047

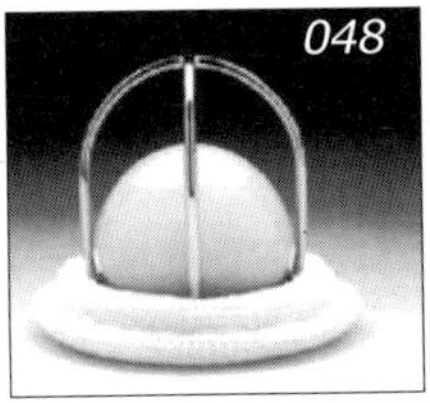

048

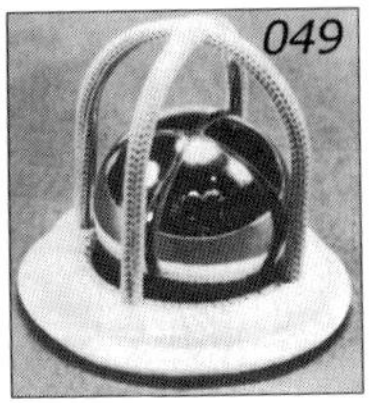

049

alterations such as a composite seat *(Figure 050)* with metal studs and cloth (Models 6310/2310) and a metallic track *(Figure 051)* along the inner surface of the struts (Models 6400/ 2400). These models were available from 1970 to 1976 and 1972 to 1980, respectively.

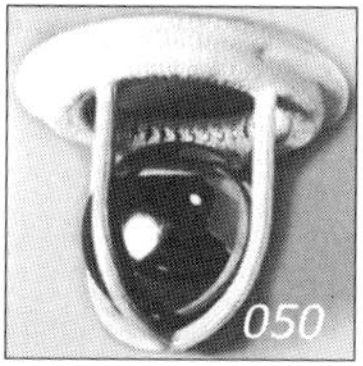
050

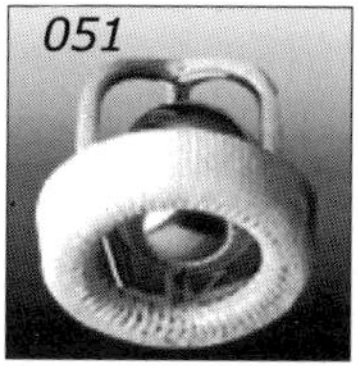
051

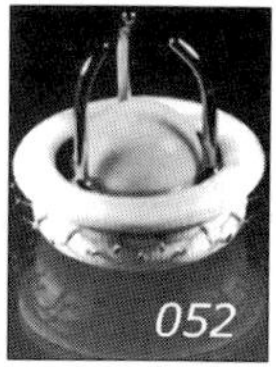
052

In 1961 (first human implant 1962), Dr George J Magovern of the University of Pittsburgh School of Medicine, along with Cromie, developed a heart valve prosthesis designed to be implanted without using sutures.[52] Originally it had a stainless steel cage with a silcone rubber ball. The rim had a string of curved metal hooks which could anchor themselves to the aorta on rotating the cage *(Figure 052)* The initial prototype did not have any cloth covering *(Figure 053)*. A rotator handle *(Figure 054)* facilitated the release of the anchoring hooks. Although the chief advantage of this valve was a significantly reduced cross-clamp time, it had an unacceptable incidence of postoperative heart block.[53] In 1964, Mr George Siposs of the Edwards Laboratories, along with Starr and others, designed the Starr-Edwards True-Pierce rotary pin

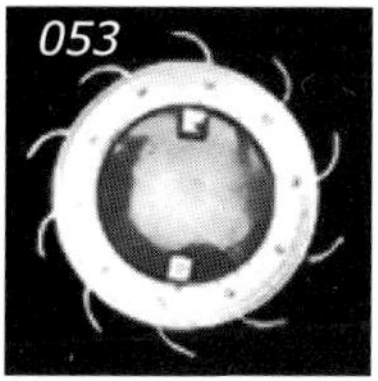
053

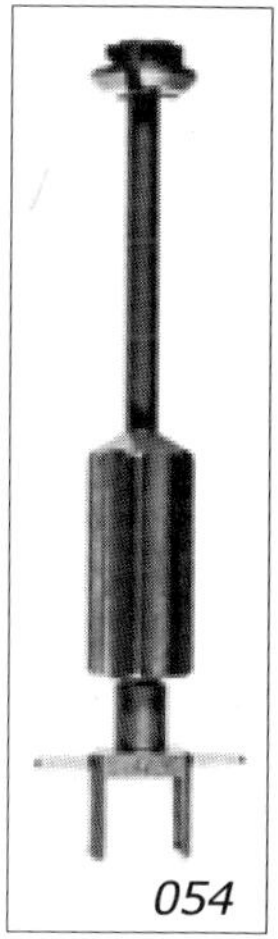
054

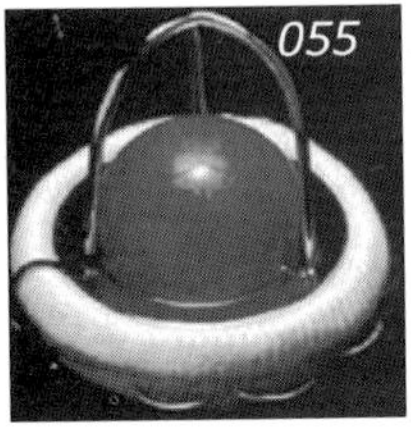

valve (US Patent 3371352 of 1968). It had a cage ring and a seat ring which could rotate coaxially and were held together by pins housed in radial holes in the cage ring *(Figure 055)*. Dr Arthur C Beall of the Baylor College of Medicine, Houston

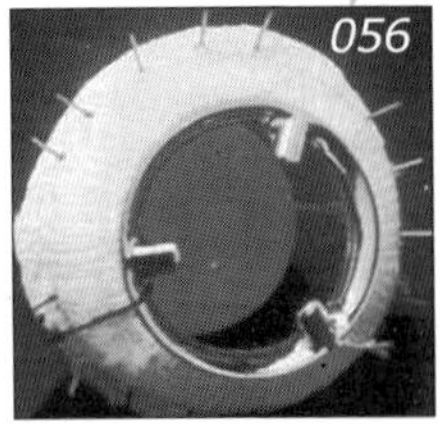

joined Siposs in designing the Beall–Edwards spring pin valve. It had retracted pins which were held by 'parachute strings' to an insertion handle and got released when a single string was cut (*Figure 056)*. Neither was clinically tried.

In 1964, Dr Edward A Smeloff and his colleagues at the Sutter Hospitals, Sacramento, California unveiled a ball and cage valve designed to provide better haemodynamics. It had a three–strut open cage on either side, the inflow cage being lesser in depth, carved out of a single block of titanium. The valve *(Figure 057)* had a Teflon sewing ring.[54] The silicone rubber ball was developed with mild–cure process by the Cutter Laboratories and the prosthesis came to be known as the Smeloff–Cutter valve

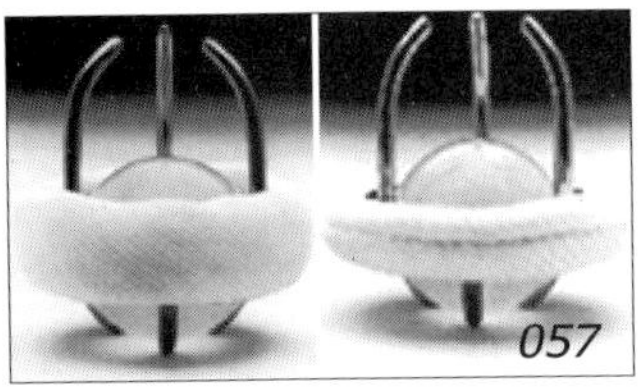

or the Smeloff-SCDK-Cutter valve.[55] Smeloff's associate in this project was Dr Robert Cartwright, credited with the first combined aortic and mitral valve replacement performed on 1 November 1961. He used Starr–Edwards valves in both the positions. Interestingly, he gained access

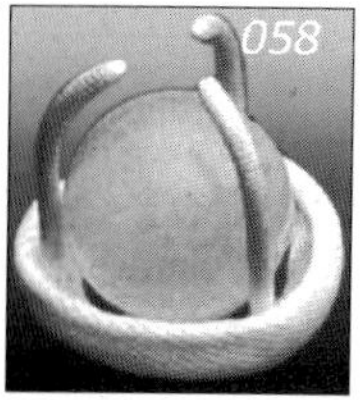

to the aortic valve via the left atrium and ventricle after excising the anterior mitral leaflet.[41]

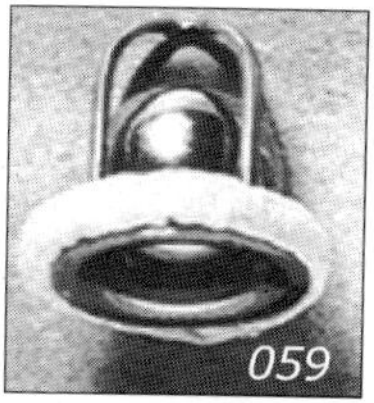

The Braunwald–Cutter valve designed by Braunwald in 1966 had an open cage design *(Figure 058)*. It had a titanium housing and struts. The housing was covered with, and the sewing ring made from ultrathin polypropylene mesh. The struts were covered with knitted Dacron tubing and the ball was similar to the one used by Smeloff. The first human implantation was done in 1968 and the device was deployed at both aortic and mitral positions.

Drs M Servelle and G Arbonville[56] of St Michel Hôpital, Paris, introduced an all–metal (stainless steel) ball and cage valve *(Figure 059)* for both aortic and mitral positions. It had a Teflon sewing ring attached to the base of the cage by a stainless steel collar held by a screw. Their device was put to clinical use in 1964, but not much has been heard of it since. In 1965, Mr Henry G de Laszlo of Cambridge, UK, associated with the Societe le Carbone-Lorraine was one of the earliest to propose the use

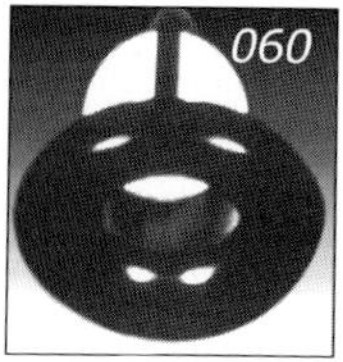

of carbonaceous materials for the fabrication of prosthetic valves *(Figure 060)*. Dr Michael DeBakey of the Baylor College of Medicine, Houston and Cromie developed the Debakey–Surgitool caged ball prosthesis *(Figure 061)* mainly for the aortic position with the collaboration of Mr Jack Bokros who introduced a pyrolytic carbon called Pyrolite. The cage and the ball were made from titanium. The titanium housing was covered with Dacron velour, though for some time an ultrahigh molecular weight polyethylene sewing ring was tried. The hollow ball surface was coated with a Pyrolite silicone compound and a radio-opaque tungsten screen was applied on its inner surface.[57] Cromie joined Drs Denton Cooley and Domingo Liotta[58] from the same place to design the Cooley–Liotta–Cromie ball and cage valve *(Figure 062)*, which had a titanium ball and a totally Dacron velour–clad cage.

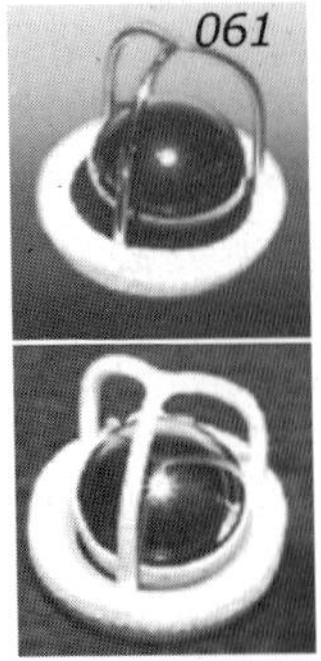
061

Self-retaining disc valves

Human ingenuity, propped by motivation and perseverance, manifested in several other concepts in prosthetic heart valves. Scientists, notably Mr CC Goosen, from the Council of Scientific and Industrial Research, Cape Town, gave shape to Barnard's concept of a self-retaining lenticular valve.[59] In its original form, designed for the mitral valve, the device had a fenestrated stainless steel ring and a slightly raised suspension bar with a loop at its end. The ring was covered with an

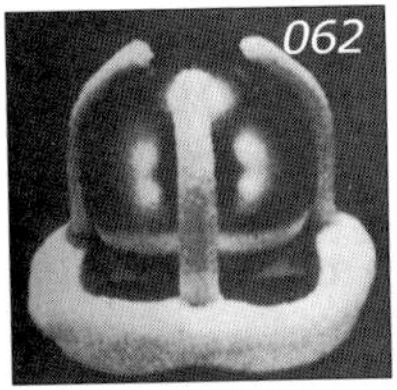
062

Ivalon (compressed polyvinyl sponge) sewing ring. The Silastic disc had a stem which would pass through the loop, a cross-bar at its end preventing its escape *(Figure 063)*. The design underwent a number of modifications according to the position it was

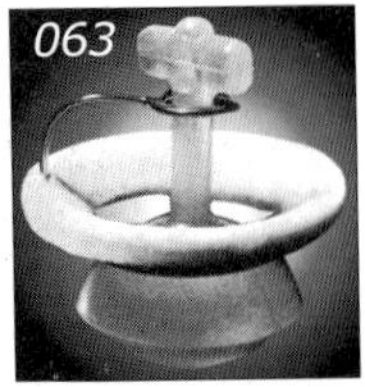
063

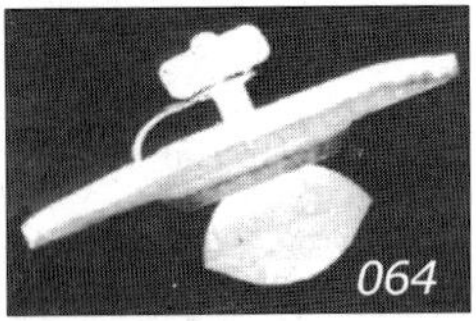

intended for.[60] A flatter disc was used for the tricuspid valve *(Figure 064)* whereas the aortic model had two looped suspension bars at either end *(Figure 065)* so

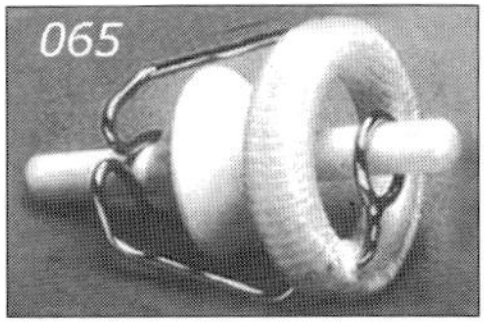

that the cross-bar could be dispensed with. Christened the University of Cape Town prosthesis, it was popularly known as the Barnard-Goosen valve and had been briefly used at the Mayo Clinic, distributed in the USA by USCI under the name Lancer.

Another variety of self-retaining disc valve was developed by Dr DG Melrose and associates[61] from the Postgraduate Medical School at Hammersmith. Their device comprised a moulded polypropylene lenticular disc with 'feet' which would act as a restraining device against the valve housing *(Figure 066)*. Independent design modifications, with eccentric disc excursion aimed at an optimally directed blood flow, were attempted by two co-workers. Dr JB Flege incorporated steel retaining pins loosely secured within a plastic ring, which gave the device the appearance of a flap valve *(Figure 067)*. Dr FR Alvarez Diaz simply repositioned the self-retaining 'feet' and modified the ring

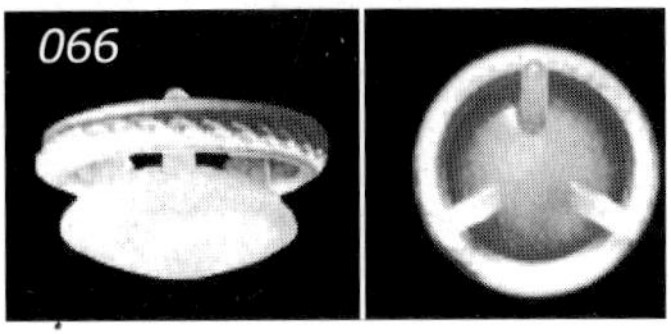

design *(Figure 068)*. Melrose's valve, which became popular as the Hammersmith valve, underwent further design changes[62] which were

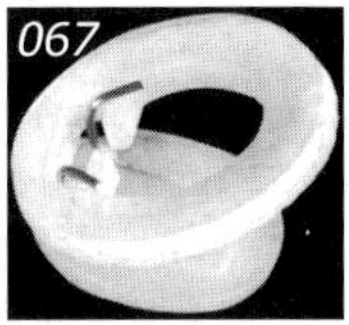

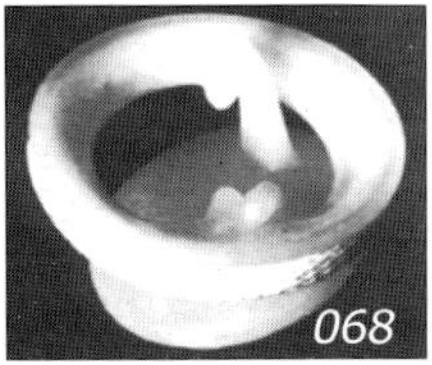
068

labelled Hammersmith Mark II *(Figure 069)* and Mark III *(Figure 070)*. Flege[63] had also designed a dual-occluder aortic valve *(Figure 071)* on similar lines. Other designs of self-retaining or hinged-disc valves experimented with included the vulcanised silicone disc valve *(Figure 072)* designed by Drs Frederick S Cross, Richard D Jones and associates, from the St Luke's Hospital, Cleveland;[64] from the Templety Health Sciences Centre, Philadelphia, Dr Julio C Davila's valve[65] with a machined or moulded polypropylene occluder suspended in a Dacron-covered Vitallium ring *(Figure 073)*; and van der Spuy's 'toilet-seat' heart valve *(Figure 074)*.

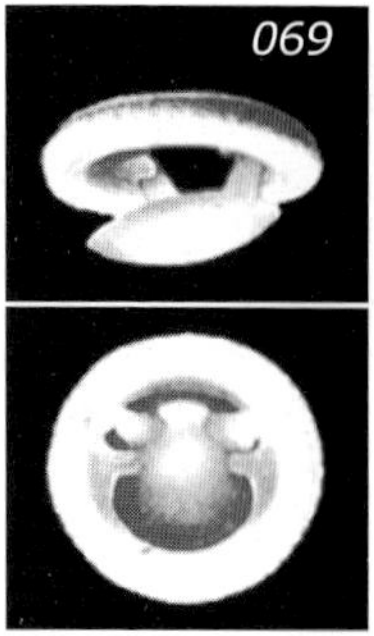
069

Caged disc valves

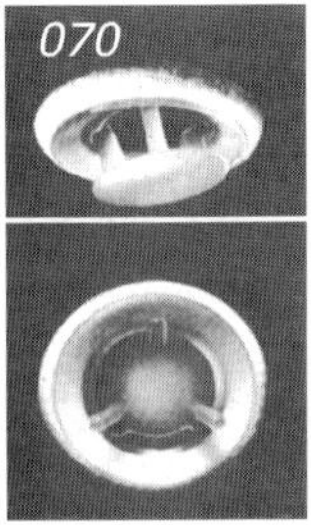
070

A number of investigators made efforts to convert the high-profile caged ball into a low-profile one by substituting a disc for the ball. These designs reduced the chance of having a mitral valve disc impinge upon the structures in the left ventricle; but such a change neither

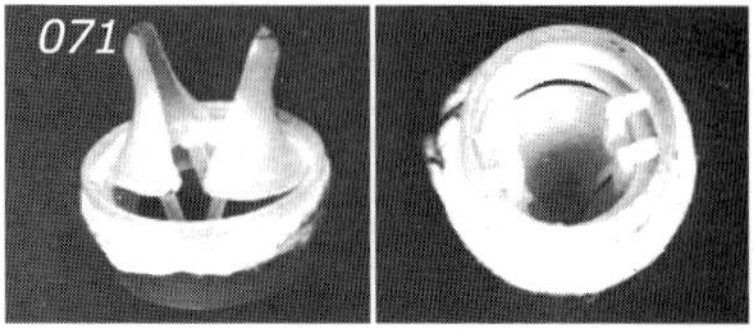
071

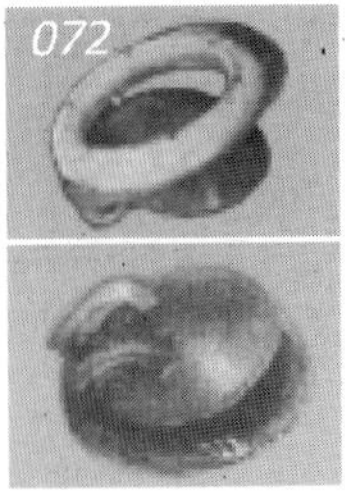
072

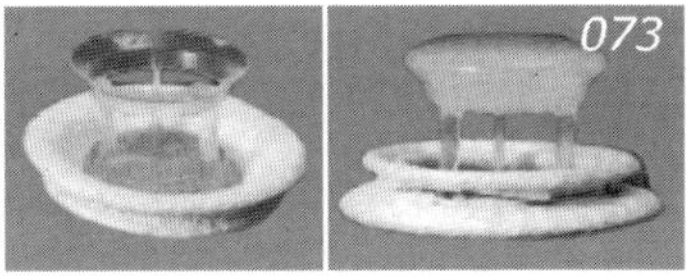
073

improved the device haemodynamics nor lessened the risk of thromboembolism.

In 1963, Kay and Suzuki developed their disc valve with a large fulcrum area *(Figure 075)* for both mitral and aortic positions.[66] A closed-cage polypropylene valve with a 'spheroidal' disc made from polypropylene covered with silicone rubber *(Figure 076)* was fabricated for Hufnagel and his associate Dr Peter W Conrad by Brunswick Mfg Co. Interestingly, the product was manufactured in nine different sizes, ranging between 12 mm and 27.5 mm, lending it the versatility of size and location of implantation. An open post version *(Figure 077)* of the same was also fabricated and was coated with Hepacone (silcone and heparin). Dr Kirkley R Williams and co-workers, from the University of Pennsylvania School of Medicine, Philadelphia, designed a caged, stainless steel-disc mitral valve prosthesis *(Figure 078)*. The disc was made from very thin, polished stainless steel. The convex side of the concavo-convex disc faced the left ventricle. The metal cage had a fabric sewing ring and four struts.[67]

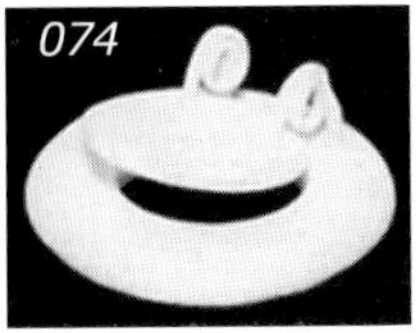
074

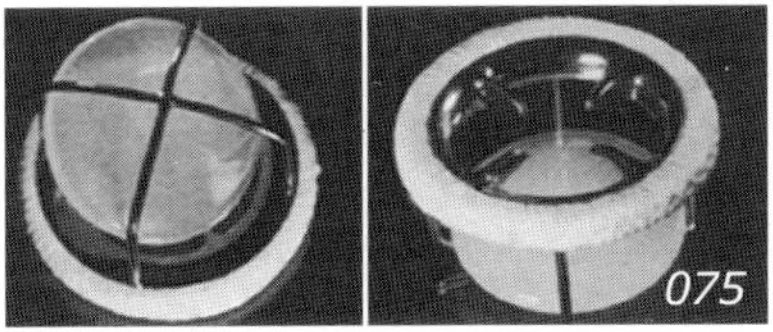
075

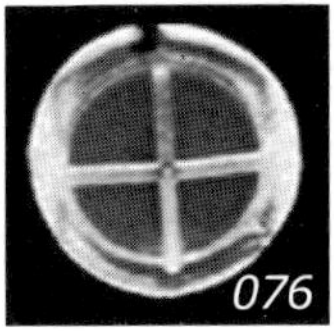
076

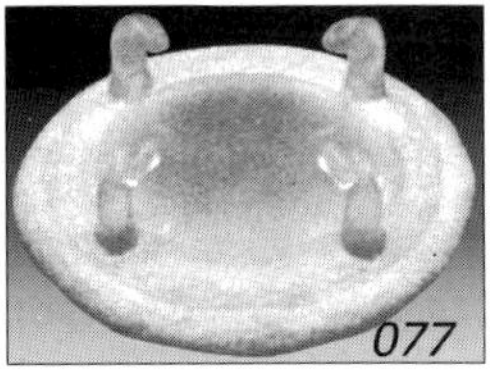

077

In 1964, Drs Antolio B Cruz and Robert L Kaster from Lillehei's group showcased a caged meniscus valve, which proved to be a landmark design for future generations of heart valve prostheses.[68] This valve consisted of a free–floating, meniscus–shaped disc of Teflon or Silastic which was encased in a cage made out of four stainless steel–vitallium struts seated upon a base of the same material *(Figure 079)*. The disc had a range of angular displacement up to 80 to 85 degrees while pivoting on one side. This greatly reduced the resistance to blood flow. The groove in the metal base was meant for a sewing cuff of woven Teflon. This served as a sewing ring for implantation of the device.

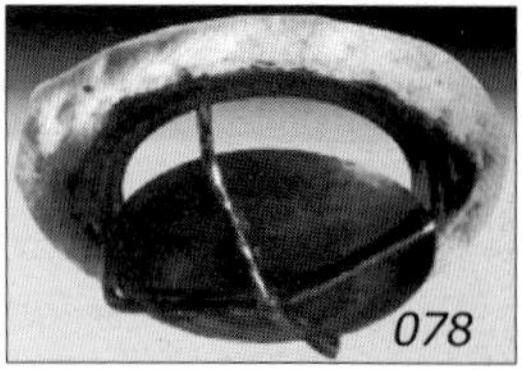

078

In 1964, Dr Jerome Harold Kay from the St Vincent's Hospital and University of South California School of Medicine, Los Angeles, California teamed up with Mr Donald Shiley, former Chief Engineer at the Edwards Laboratories, who had just launched his own enterprise, the Shiley Laboratories, Inc in Santa Ana, California. Together they experimented with a low–profile atrioventricular valve prosthesis.[69] The device comprised a Stellite cage with two parallel Stellite struts, and a Silastic disc

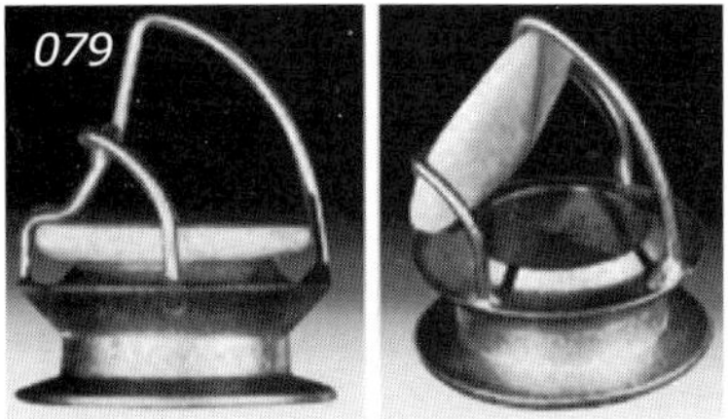

079

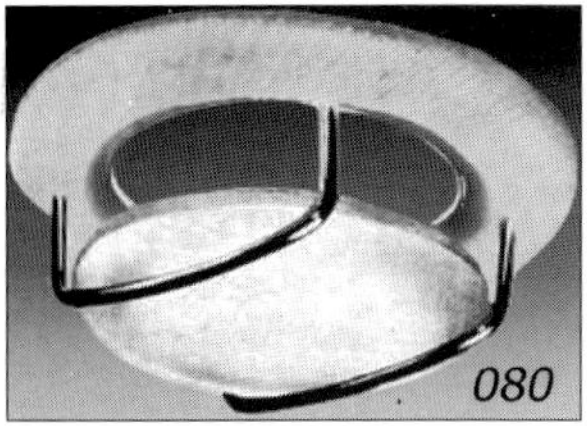

(Figure 080). Also tried in the course of its development were Haynes-25 alloy for the cage and Delrin for the disc. The Kay-Shiley valve was first put to clinical use in 1965 for tricuspid valve replacement in a case of Ebstein's anomaly. The basic design underwent several offbeat modifications such as incorporation of single *(Figure 081)* and double *(Figure 082)* muscle guards to prevent disc movement interference by the ventricular wall. In 1966, Dr Ahmad Nakib, working with Lillehei, designed an all-titanium toroidal disc valve *(Figure 083)*, manufactured by Washington Scientific Industries, which had provision for central as well as peripheral flow.[70] Cross and Jones had a low-profile valve fabricated by Pemco, Inc. The device had a titanium ring and cage, a woven Teflon sewing flange (later changed to Dacron), and a lenticular silicone rubber disc reinforced with a thin ring of titanium *(Figure 084)*. In a later model, the disc was forged

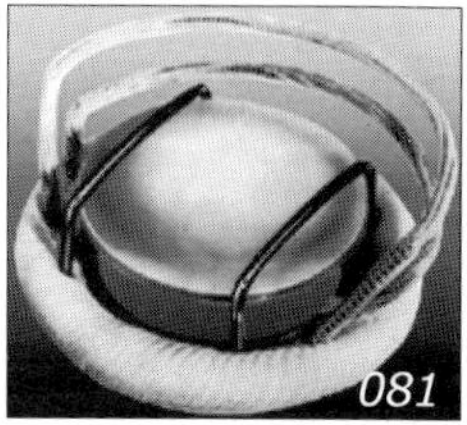

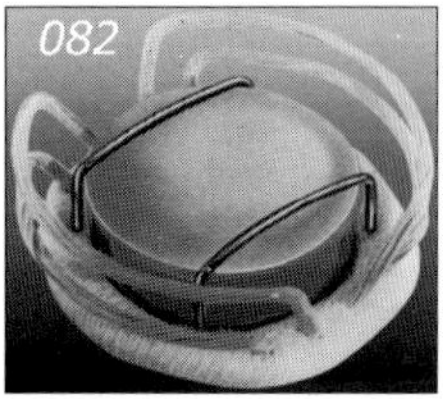

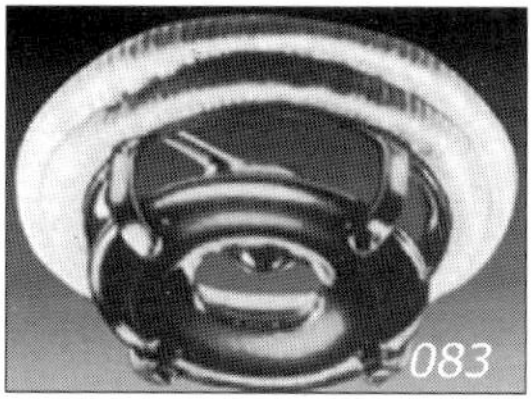

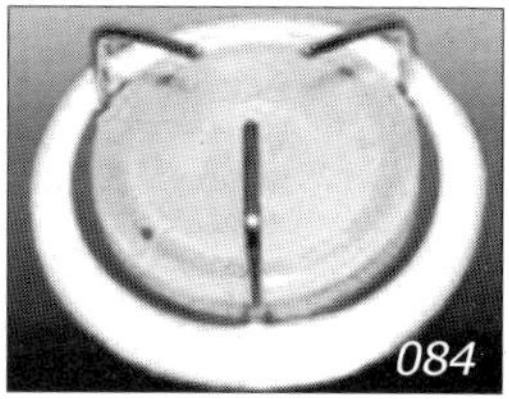

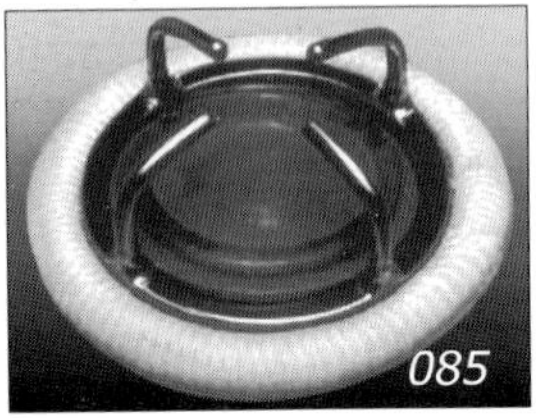

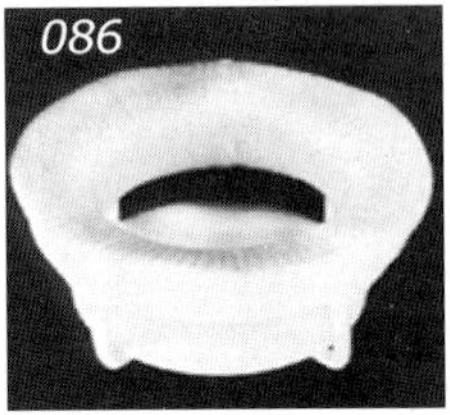

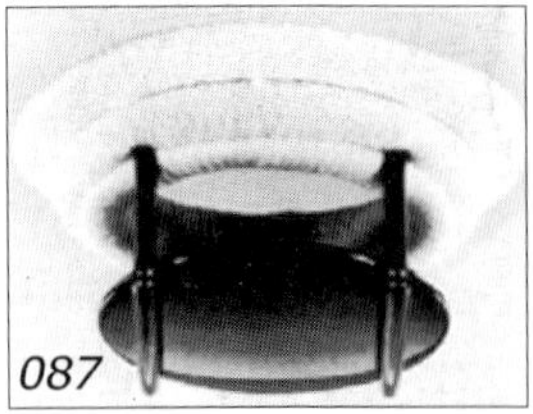

from titanium *(Figure 085)*.[71] Drs Beall, Jr, Robert D Bloodwell and Liotta, from the then DeBakey–Cooley team at Baylor, teamed up with Cromie of Surgitool to create the Beall–Surgitool Model 102 *(Figure 086)* in 1967. It was a Dacron velour–covered, Teflon disc low-profile valve whose titanium cage had two arch-like struts coated with Teflon.[72] This design underwent several modifications culminating in Model 106 *(Figure 087)* incorporating a Pyrolyte disc and struts coated with the same material. A turtle–neck ring model had also been tried. *(Figure 088)* The same year, Cromie was once again the member of a valve team, this time to manufacture a caged–disc mitral prosthesis designed by Harken.[73] The

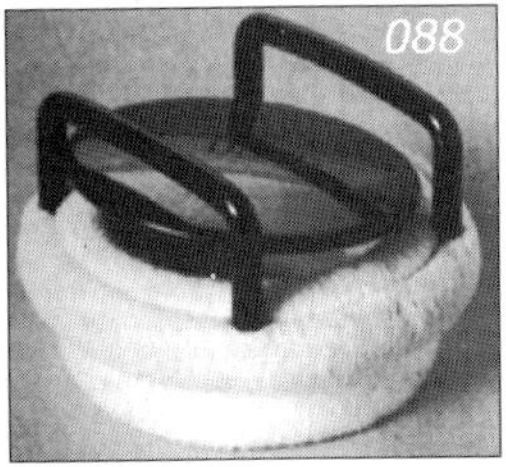

valve had a titanium cage with four thin struts crossing in the middle *(Figure 089)*. It had a silicone disc and a Dacron sewing ring. The Starr and Edwards team also released its own version of the caged-disc valve,

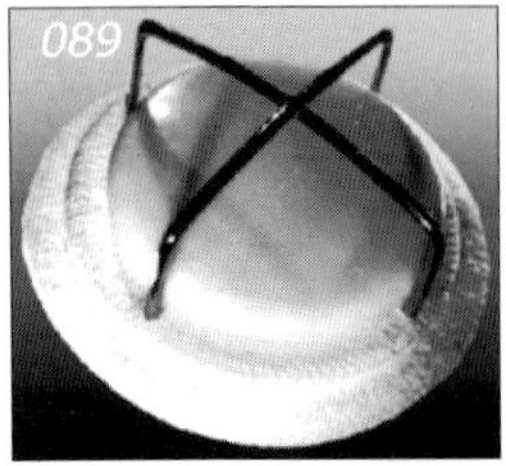

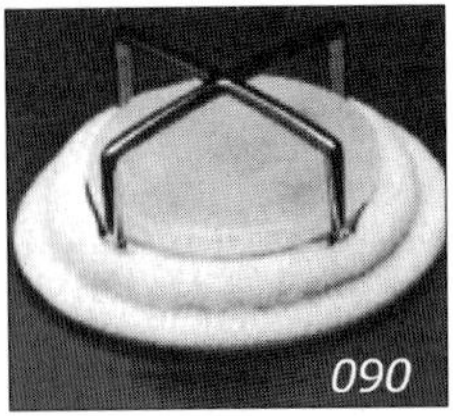

090

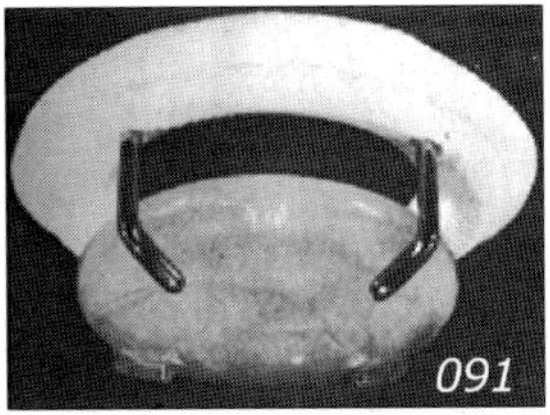

091

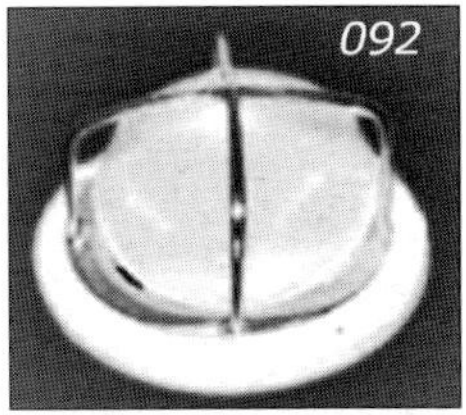

092

named Model 6500 in 1968.[74] It had a hollow Stellite-21 poppet in a four-strut closed cage of the same material, and a Teflon sewing ring. In an improved version (Model 6520) the disc material was changed to ultrahigh molecular weight polyethylene (Hifax), now marketed as with an embedded titanium ring *(Figure 090)*. Other disc and cage valve prostheses included the Cooley-Bloodwell-Cutter valve with an open *(Figure 091)* and a closed cage *(Figure 092)*, the Cooley-Cutter valve[75] with a biconical Pyrolyte disc *(Figure 093)*, the University of Stellenbosch disc valve *(Figure 094)* designed by Dr PM Barnard (not related to Christiaan Barnard)[76] from South Africa and the Servelle metallic disc valves *(Figure 095)*.

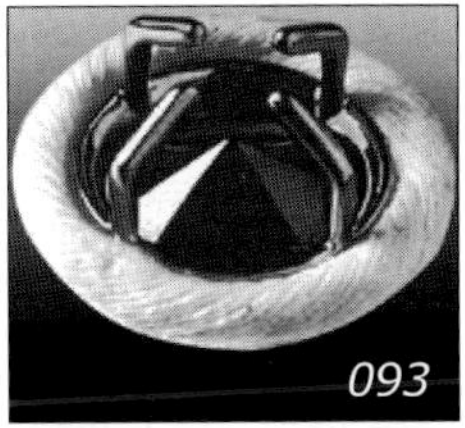

093

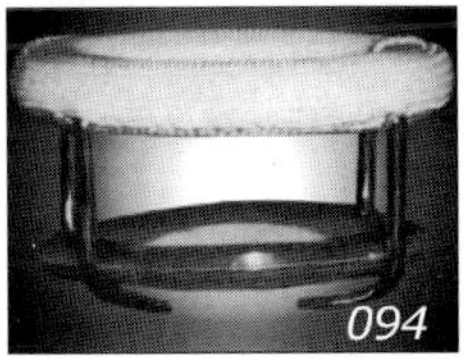

094

Tilting disc valves

The concept of a tilting disc valve emerged out of the need for prostheses which were less bulky and haemodynamically superior to the

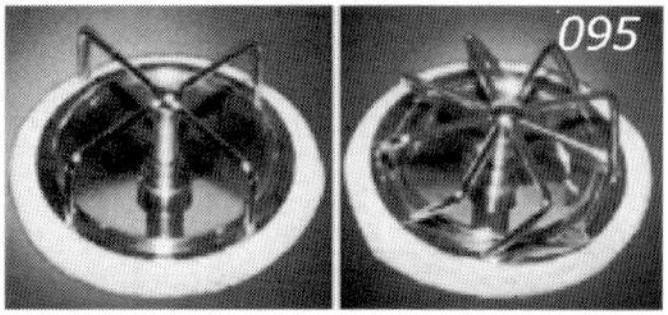

095

existent caged-poppet varieties. A flat pivoting disc mounted on hinges was expected to dramatically reduce the cross-sectional area when open.

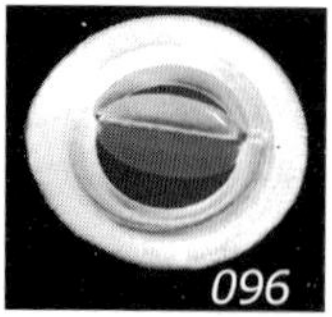

096

Drs WS Pierce, DM Behrendt and AG Morrow of the National Heart and Lung Institute, designed a tilting disc valve *(Figure 096)* on an experimental basis in 1966.[77] Although it had only one moving disc, it was patented as a 'pivoted butterfly' type heart valve (US Patent 3448465 of 1969). Also in 1966, Dr Juro Wada of the Sapporo Medical College Hospital, had the design concept of a pivoting, hingeless, tilting disc valve. He got it fabricated by Cutter Biomedicals.[78] The device consisted of a metallic ring of titanium, an occluder of a solid, hard Teflon/Halon, and a sewing ring of Teflon. Two notches on the occluder were engaged by two claws on opposite sides of the internal surface of the metallic ring, allowing opening and closing *(Figure 097)*. The first total artificial heart implanted in 1969 by Denton Cooley was equipped with four Wada-Cutter valves.

Miscellaneous valve designs

Several other innovative valve designs emanated during this probational phase of heart valve development. In 1959, Kolff's group[79] designed a flexible-leaflet cylindroid polyurethane valve with

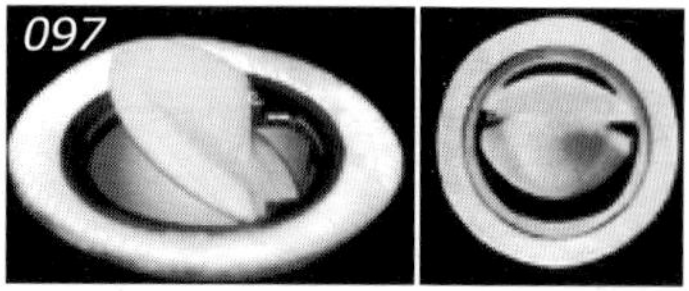

097

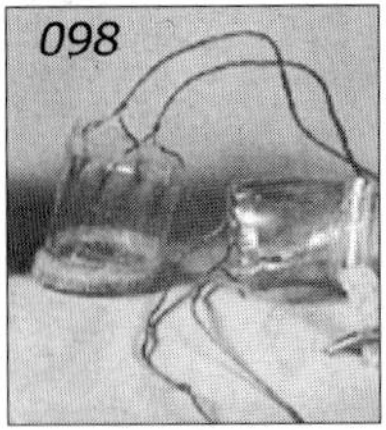

098

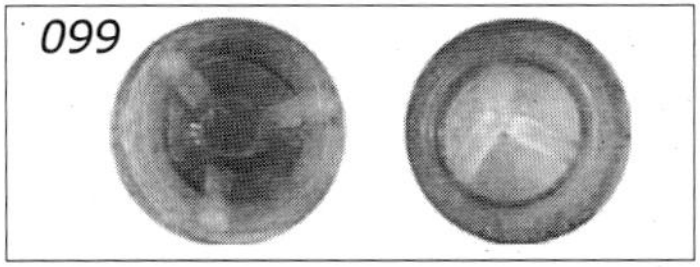

099

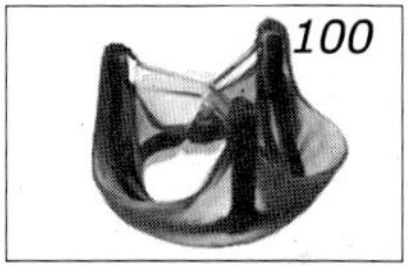

100

braided chordae *(Figure 098)* with the express objective of keeping thrombus formation at bay, but in vain. In 1963, Dr Richard W Ernst of the University of Texas Southwestern Medical School, Dallas, Texas and Mr Harry D Stokes, a bio-engineer from the same university,[80] had experimented with a conical mitral valve prosthesis made of three injection-moulded Silastic leaflets incorporated into a frame of the same material *(Figure 099)*. Dr Hitoshi Mohri and colleagues[81] fabricated die-injected, trileaflet Silastic aortic valves *(Figure 100)* and put them through durability tests. Dr Hillary H Timmis[82] of the University of Pennsylvania School of Medicine, Philadelphia described an ingeniously designed spring-valve cuspal prosthesis *(Figure 101)*; A Silastic-Dacron mesh valve with a cuff of Ivalon was fabricated by Dr William G Esmond[83] and associates from the University Hospital of Maryland, Baltimore. The designed configurations were with *(Figure 102)* and without *(Figure 103)* chordal appendages.

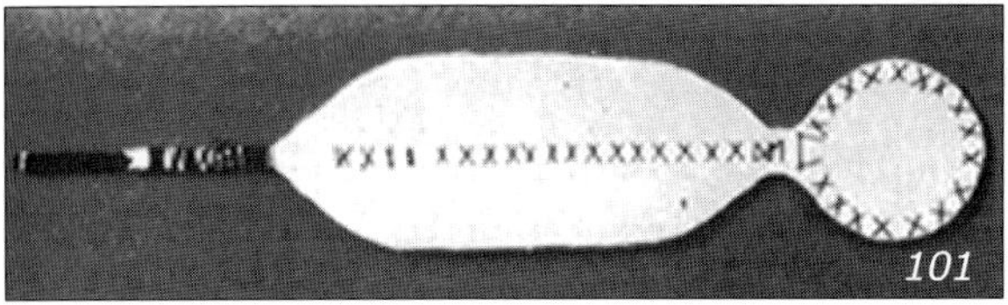

101

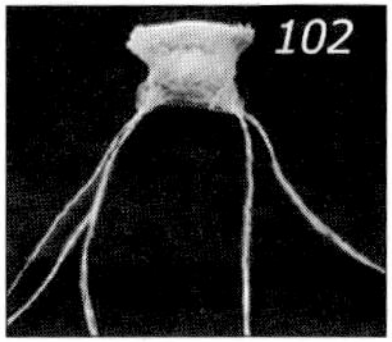

102

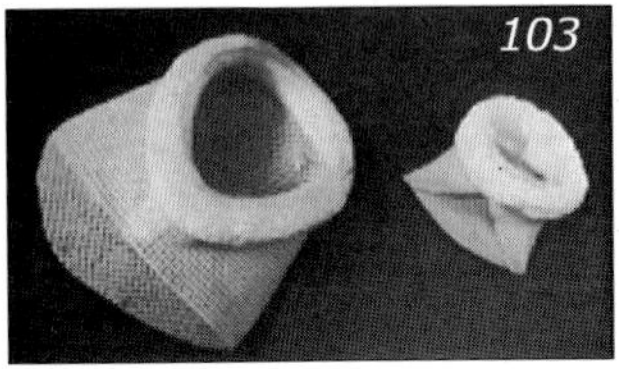

103

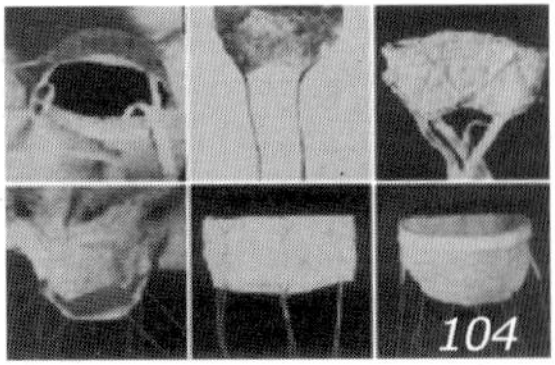

104

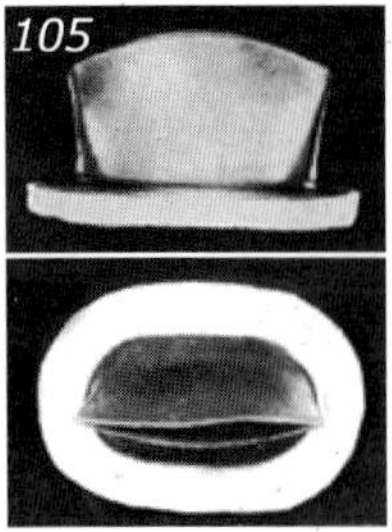

105

Several other cuspal prototypes *(Figure 104)* were also experimented with.[84,85] Some creations which evinced considerable interest were a valve by Dr David M Long Jr,[86] an associate of Lillehei *(Figure 105)*; one by Drs William H Muller Jr and James B Littlefield[87] of the University of Virginia School of Medicine, Charlottesville *(Figure 106)*; duPlessis–Morrow's Teflon valve *(Figure 107)*; and certain Dacron–Silastic models fabricated by Hufnagel *(Figure 108)*. Dr Karl William Edmark, Jr of the University of Washington Medical Center, Seattle had designed (US Patent 3113586 of 1963) a silastic valve in the shape of an electric desk fan *(Figure 109)*. Drs Robert C Malowney and Bruce C Paton[88] from the University of Colorado School of Medicine, Denver introduced a silastic monocusp mitral prosthesis which

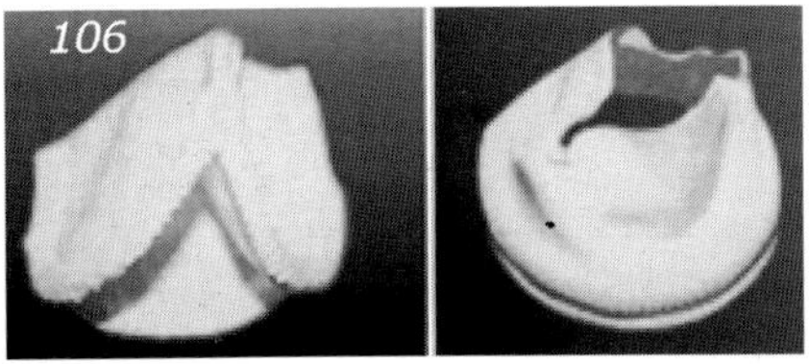

106

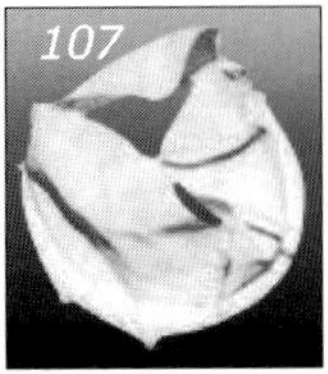

107

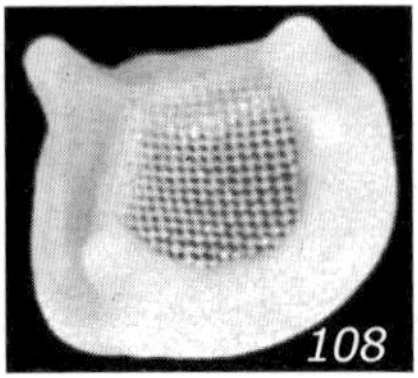

108

resembled a snuff-box *(Figure 110)*. The Edwards Laboratories had manufactured several prototypes of 'central flow' cloth–covered Silastic valves *(Figure 111)*.

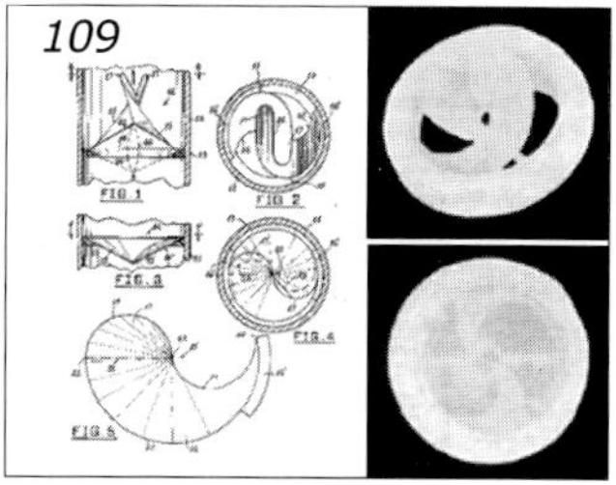

109

In the course of evolution of heart valve prostheses, several other prosthetic valve designs were conceived but perhaps failed to progress beyond the artist's canvas. Not much data could be gleaned about these designs; yet they reflected the spirit of human ingenuity striving to ameliorate human distress. Some of these concepts/designs were patented, such as an innovative magnetic hinge mechanism patented by Dr B Goott and others (US Patent 3370305 of 1968); Mr Jack C Bokros' tilting disc *(Figure 112)* prosthesis (US Patent 3546711 of 1970); an umbrella-like flexible wall *(Figure 113)* heart valve designed by Dr RD Kischer (US Patent 3548417 of 1970); A prosthetic valve with cylindrical housing, rectangular opening and triangular flaps controlled by a floating ball *(Figure 114)* patented by Dr Richard K Rapp (US Patent 3689942 of 1972); Cooley, Liotta and Dr Paul Kahn's bicuspid *(Figure 115)*

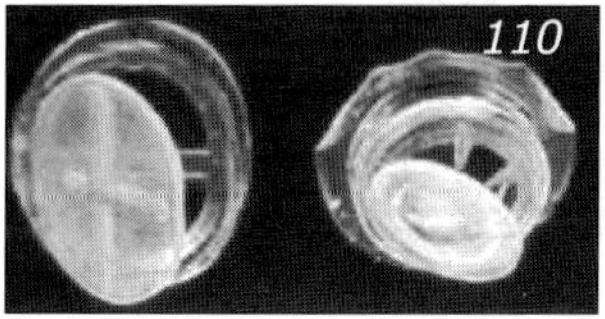

110

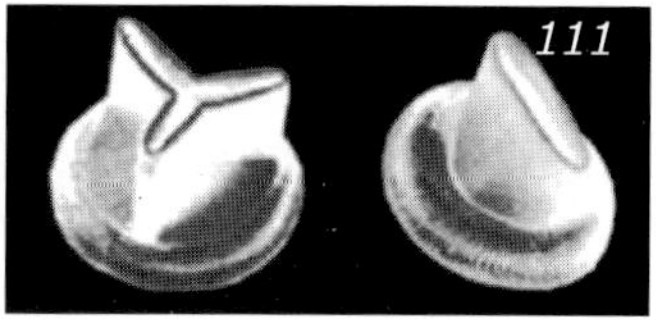

111

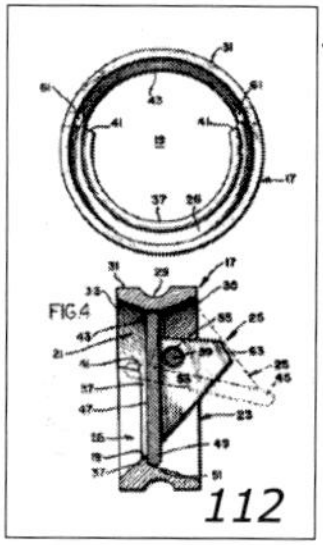

112

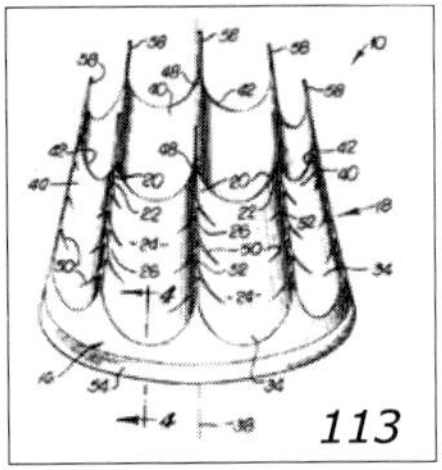
113

fascia lata valve (US Patent 3739402 of 1973), Dr Francis W Child's pivoting disc prosthesis (US Patent 3835475 of 1974); Dr Ahmad A Nakib's free-floating double disc *(Figure 116)* valve (US Patent 3903548 of 1975); and Dr Bruce E Fettel's tilting disc prosthesis with an arcuate occluder (US Patent 4057857 of 1977). A number of innovative spring-based Japanese valves were also showcased *(Figure 117)*.

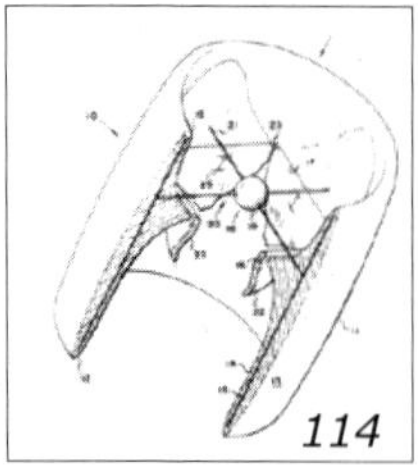
114

Biomaterials as valve substitutes

Aortic valve allografts

In 1962, Drs Alfred J Gunning and Carlos G Duran of the Radcliffe Infirmary, Oxford, pioneered aortic homograft replacement in the subcoronary position *(Figure 118)*. They practised the technique of suitably fashioning aortic valves harvested from donor cadavers and

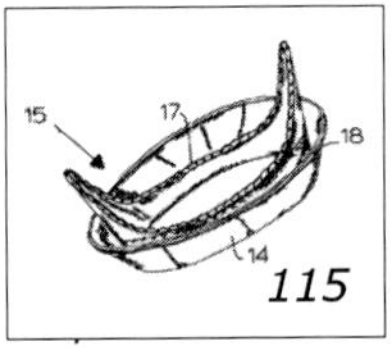
115

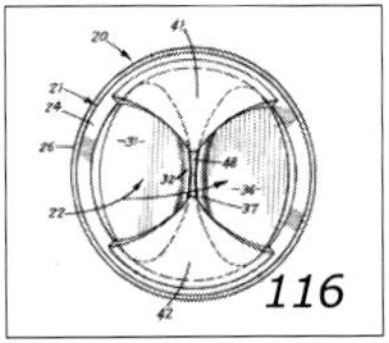
116

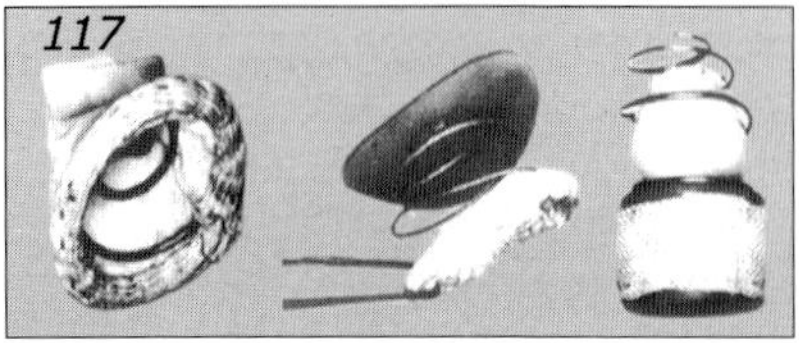
117

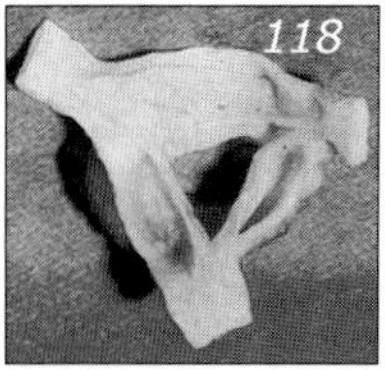

inserting them in the subcoronary position in cadaveric recepients. The efficacy of the procedure was successfully demonstrated in a pulse duplicator.[89] In the same year, Mr Donald Nixon Ross of the National Heart and Guy's Hospitals, London[90] and Dr Brian Gerald Barratt–Boyes of the Green Lane Hospital, Auckland[91] performed successful orthotopic homograft implantations. Subsequently, both were decorated with knignthood. The era of stentless valves had begun.

With rising concerns about the sterilisation and viability of these valves, several research projects were initiated. Options tried for sterilisation included ethylene oxide, betapropriolactone and gamma-irradiation. Valve storage in tissue-friendly, antibiotic-rich hypothermic media became the norm. The process of freeze-drying, as a precursor to cryopreservation, was introduced.[92] Ross, Barratt–Boyes and Shumway succeeded in sustaining homograft aortic valve implantation programmes at their respective centres. The insertion of homografts was facilitated by mounting them on a rigid Teflon–covered stent fabricated by Cutter Laboratories. On 23 March 1962, Dr RO Heimbecker and colleagues at the Toronto General Hospital created history by replacing the heavily calcified, stenotic mitral valve of a 46–year–old man with an aortic homograft.[93] Dr William W Angell, an associate of Shumway,[94] and Dr MA Rogers (Wentworth Hospital, University of Natal, South Africa)[95] were among the first to report the use of stent-mounted aortic homografts *(Figure 119)* for mitral valve replacement.

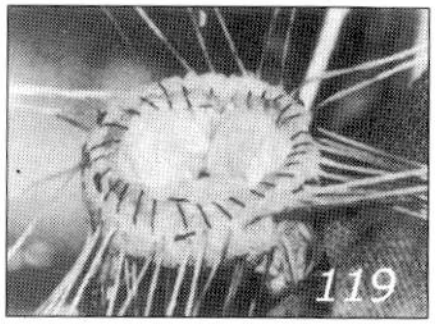

Porcine valve xenografts

In 1965, Drs Jean–Paul Binet, Alain Frédéric Carpentier, and colleagues at the Centre Chirurgical Marie-Lannelongue in Paris, implanted for the first time ever, an aortic valve xenograft in a human subject from a nonhuman (porcine) source.[96] A year later, Dr Mark F O'Brien[97] of the Prince Charles Hospital, Brisbane, Australia reported his work with bovine and porcine heterografts. This triggered similar efforts in several countries, along with the search for appropriate methods to sterilise these grafts and reduce their antigenicity. Towards the end of the decade, Carpentier, now under Dr Charles DuBost at the Clinique de Leriche at Hôpital Bröussais in Paris, experimented with several options of xenograft preservation and finally initiated the nomenclature of 'bioprosthesis'. This also marked the beginning of the glutaraldehyde treatment era for preservation of heterologous tissues. In 1968, Carpentier implanted the first ever glutaraldehyde-treated porcine aortic valve, mounted on a stent. Edwards Laboratories evinced interest in this valve leading to its commercial availability as the Carpentier–Edwards valve *(Figure 120)*. This valve has a flexible metal stent made from Elgiloy, a corrosion-resistant cobalt–nickel alloy. The strength and flexibility of this alloy allows the use of a thinner frame, which facilitates better flow characteristics across the device.[96]

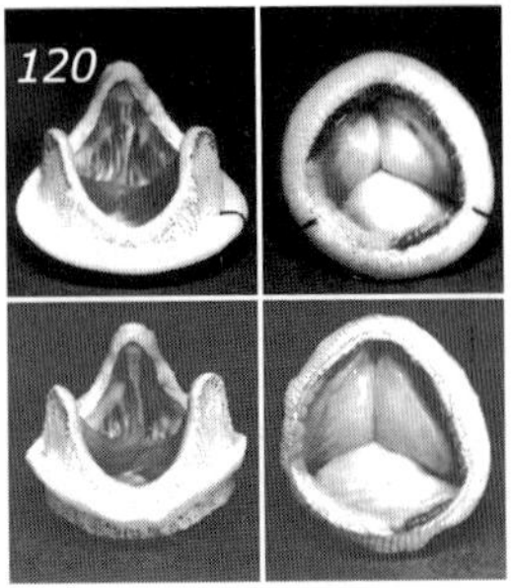

As a contemporary competitor, an Edwards Laboratories ex-worker, Mr Warren D Hancock,

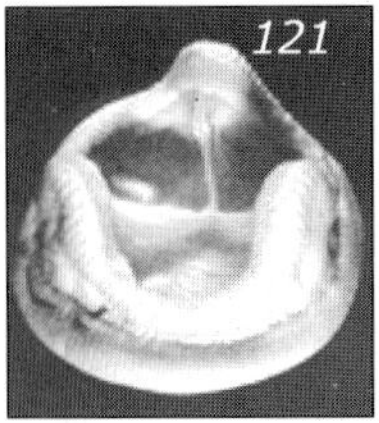

started his own company, Hancock Laboratories. He started with a formaldehyde-treated porcine valve mounted on a Dacron-covered rigid metal stent.[98] Subsequently, Dr Robert L Reis and colleagues at the National Heart and Lung Institute joined Hancock

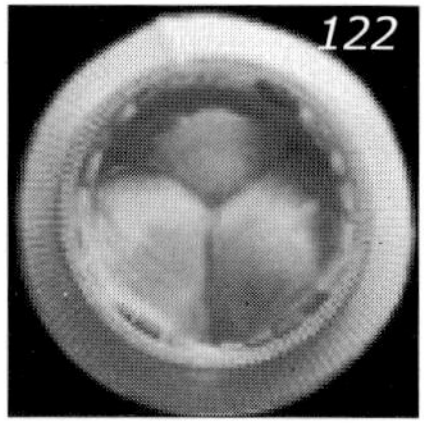

in developing a flexible stent *(Figure 121)* which had asymmetrically placed posts on a polypropylene frame with a Stellite ring covered with Dacron; and switched to glutaraldehyde as the medium of pretreatment for harvested valves.[99] Porcine aortic valves have an inherent disadvantage. The right coronary cusp is supported by an intimately attached extension of septal myocardium which hampers its mobility when used as a prosthesis. In 1967, O'Brien had introduced the concept of composite trileaflet xenografts by suturing together three noncoronary cusps. Taking the cue, Hancock started manufacturing a 'modified orifice' valve *(Figure 122)*, wherein the muscle-bound right coronary cusp was replaced by a nonmuscular cusp from another valve.[96]

Angell was another enthusiast who gave glutaraldehyde–treated xenografts a try, after his initial experience with fresh aortic valve homografts.[100] His team developed over seventy configurations *(Figure 123)* of a flexible Dacron–covered Delrin stent. These 'anatomic' stents were based on

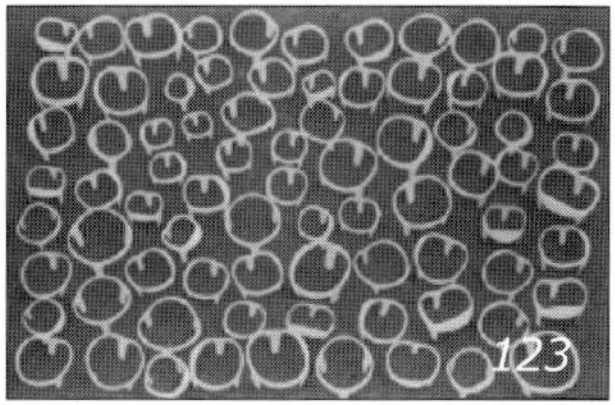

castings of porcine aortic roots to preclude any stent–valve mismatch. An eventual collaboration with Shiley Laboratories led to the creation of the Angell–Shiley bioprosthesis.

Bioprostheses from nonvalvar tissues

The difficulties and disappointments associated with available bioprosthetic devices prompted further research for newer options. Autogenous pericardium had already been tried. In 1962, Dr Ake Senning from the University Clinics, Zurich, Switzerland started using freehand, autologous fascia lata cusps and strips for diseased aortic valves.[101] Encouraged by his results, Dr Marian I Ionescu of the Leeds Infirmary, UK teamed up with Ross to design a stent-mounted fascia lata valve.[102] A scallop–shaped titanium frame covered with Dacron velour *(Figure 124)* served as a prop for suitably sized aortic as well as atrioventricular valve prostheses. Drs RT Brownlee and AK Yates[103] from the Guy's Hospital undertook clinical trials with a fascia lata mitral valve fabricated on the 'frustum' principle *(Figure 125)*. A high incidence of tissue degeneration, reported from the same institution,[104] caused interest to wane in this material. A decade later, Dr Endre Bodnar and associates[105] from the same institution described a bicuspid mitral bioprosthesis prepared by mounting glutaraldehyde–processed porcine pericardium on to the stents used by Brownlee and Yates, without much success either.

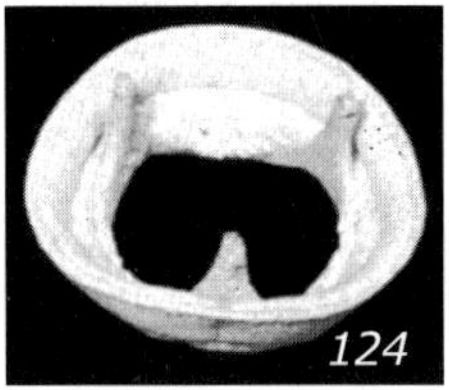

124

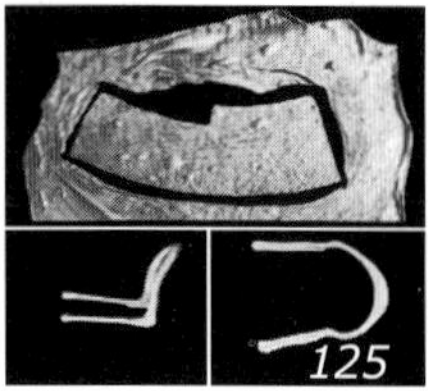

125

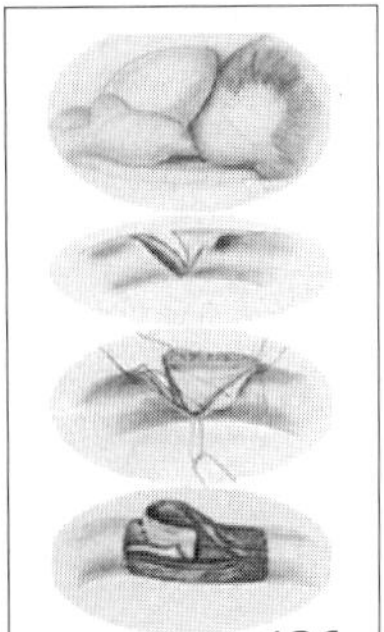

126

In 1959, Dr Karel B Absolon and colleagues from the University of Minnesota Medical School, Minneapolis, Minnesota reported the use of autologous diaphragm for the construction of a valve which was implanted into canine aortic arches.[106] Later, the same technique was applied for pulmonary valve replacement, also in dogs. The valve, constructed from the tendinous part of the diaphragm *(Figure 126)*, had a unicuspid mechanism.[107] There are no records to suggest extension of the concept to human subjects. Drs Eurcylides J Zerbini, Luiz B Puig and associates from the Heart Institute at the University of Sao Paulo Medical School, Brazil reported the use of homologous dura mater as a heart valve substitute.[108] Interestingly, the tissue, removed within 12 hours from fatal accident victims, would be preserved and sterilised in 98% glycerin for at least 12 days. A Dacron velour–covered rigid steel stent was used and only avascular portions of dura mater were selected for the valve *(Figure 127)*.

In 1971, the enormous promise held by bovine pericardium as a heart valve substitute was unfolded by Ionescu.[109] Harvested from 6– to 18–month–old calves, the material was chemically sterilised and stabilised before it was mounted on Ionescu's titanium stent.[110] The valve was manufactured in collaboration with Shiley Laboratories and was the first commercially available pericardial valve

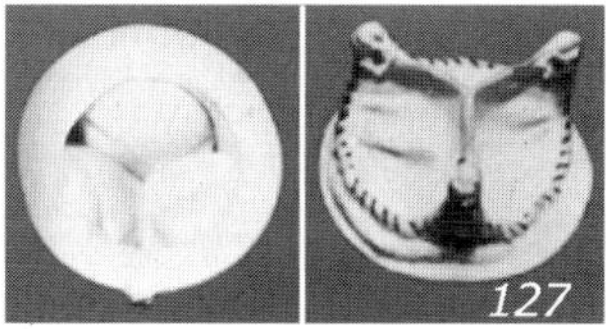

127

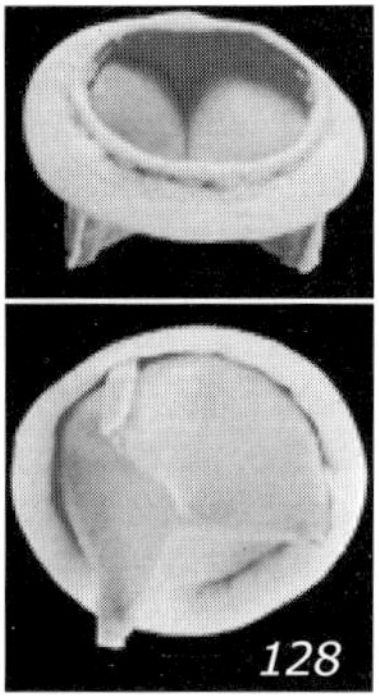

(*Figure 128*). It had excellent haemodynamics, with the average gradient substantially below that of the competing contemporary porcine valves of the time; but it registered an unacceptable rate of structural failure and was taken off the market. As a measure against such damage, Reis and Hancock had also developed a flexible stent (*Figure 129*) with symmetrically placed posts for mounting pericardium or fascia lata.[99] For a brief period, Hancock pericardial valves were introduced but were withdrawn in favour of their porcine valves. In 1976, animal experiments were also started with the Edwards pericardial xenografts that used a flexible Elgiloy stent.[111] Dr Randas J Vilela Batista[112] and associates from the Hospital Nossa Senhora das Gracas, Curitiba, Brazil tailored a strip of bovine pericardium in the shape of a patient's native valve leaflets, by superimposition, and used it as a stentless 'monopatch' valve (*Figure 130*). According to a personal communication, Dr Vilela Batista still replaces the aortic valve in this manner.

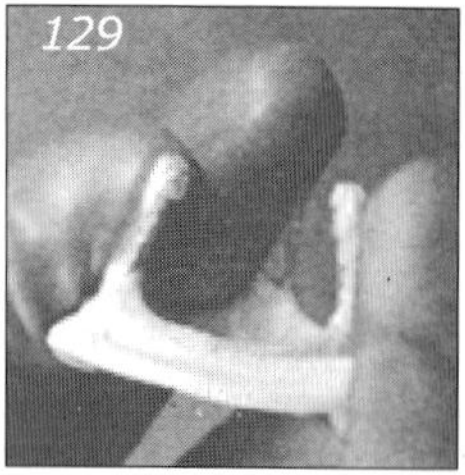

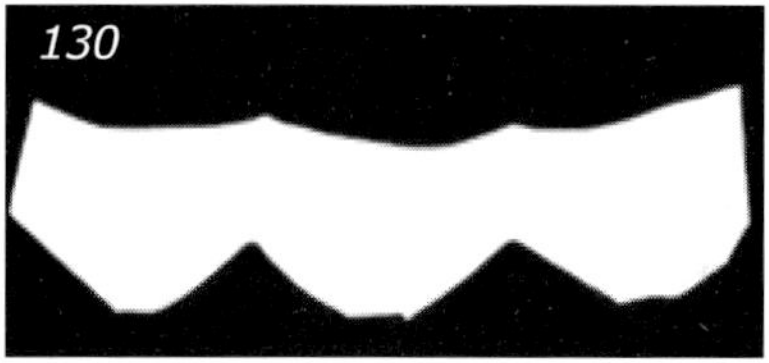

The Coeval Inventory

The last two decades of the twentieth century witnessed an impressive boom in the heart valve industry. On account of spiralling demand, compulsions of economy and the aspiration for self-reliance, many countries initiated development of indigenous heart valve prostheses. This process did not necessarily involve original research on either material or design. The prostheses manufactured and marketed during this period comprised the cohort of heart valves which are in current use. Wherever needed, modifications were made in the course of their use; some were discarded or discontinued, at times only to be revived.

Ball and cage valves

With minor modifications in the sewing ring, orifice and ball diameters and the height of the cage, Biomedica Mexicana of Mexico and Machhi Engenharia of Brazil manufactured and marketed the Biomed *(Figure 131)* and Macchi *(Figure 132)* valves, respectively. The latter had a Biolite carbon coating on the cage. James A Davidson of Germantown,

131

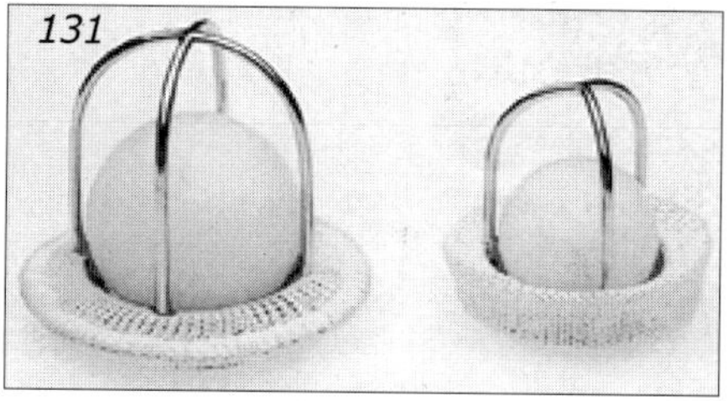

Tennessee had proposed a zirconium oxide and nitride coated caged-ball prosthesis (US Patent 5258022 of 1993). At the end, however, it was the Starr–Edwards valve (particularly Model 6120) which stood the test of time and managed to outlast its ever–evolving contemporaries.

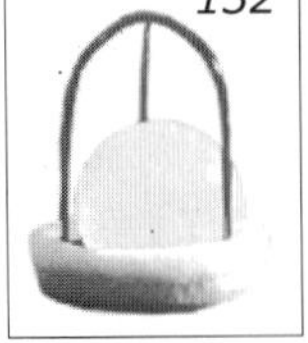

132

Bileaflet valve

The St Jude Medical mechanical prosthesis (St Jude Medical Inc, Minneapolis, Minnesota) was first implanted on 3 October 1977 by Drs Demetre Nicoloff and Robert Emery of the University of Minnesota, Minneapolis. It was fabricated on the basis of the Kalke valve and a crude design blueprinted by Nicoloff and Mr Zinon Christopher Possis, a biomedical engineer. It is a bileaflet prosthesis with pyrolytic carbon over a graphite substrate for housing and leaflets. The two semicircular leaflets open to 85°, resulting in central, near-laminar flow. The sewing cuff is usually made of double velour Dacron. Leaflets are orifice oriented and closing forces are supported by the pivot system. The pivot guards are raised above the housing in the mitral position. This minimises the intraventricular excursion of the leaflet *(Figure 133)*. In the aortic position these pivot guards protrude into the valve annulus. The original Standard St Jude Medical prosthesis was non-rotatable *(Figure 134)*. As preservation

133

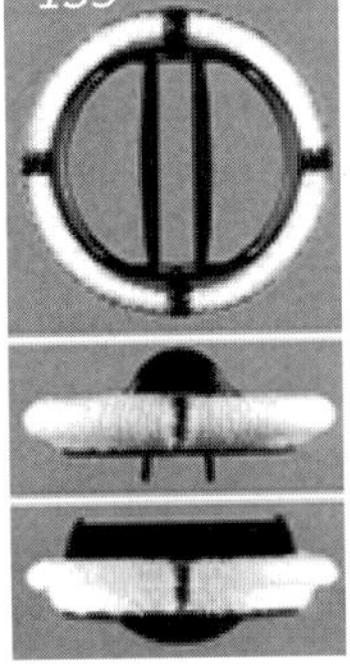

134

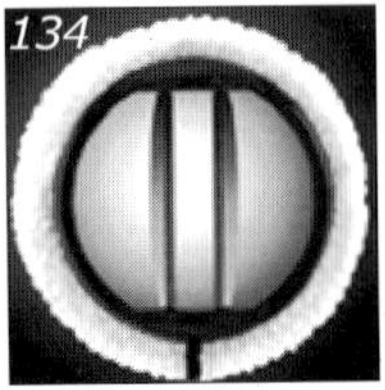

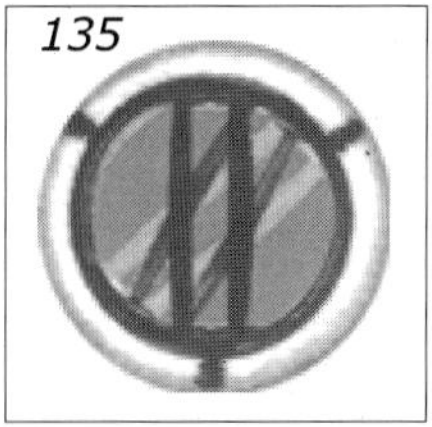

135

of mitral valve chordae became popular, a rotating mechanism was introduced in the next generation called the Masters series which also had improved radio-opacity (due to two retainer rings and a helical spring in the sewing ring) and additional

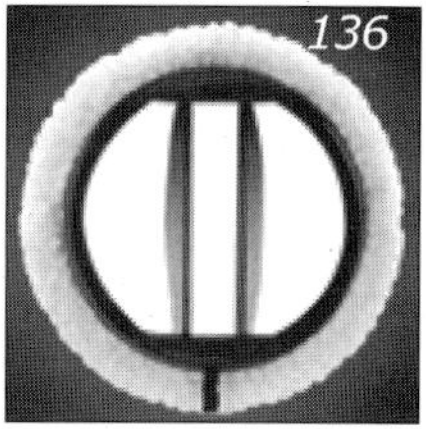

136

suture markers on the cuff *(Figure 135)*. Design modifications were incorporated — in both Standard *(Figure 136)* and Masters *(Figure 137)* configurations — to optimise their haemodynamic performance in the aortic position by providing a larger effective orifice area, minimal turbulence or stasis, and lower pressure gradients *(Figure 138)*. This concept was christened Haemodynamic Plus (HP). The sewing cuff design of the HP Series valve allows totally supra–annular placement which requires specially designed sizers to accurately gauge the native annulus size. The Silzone *(Figure 139)* valve (sewing ring impregnated with an antimicrobial agent) was introduced in 1994 with the objective of minimising the risk of endocarditis, but had to be withdrawn due to an unacceptable

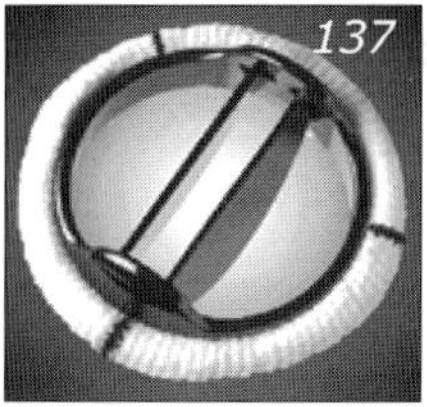

137

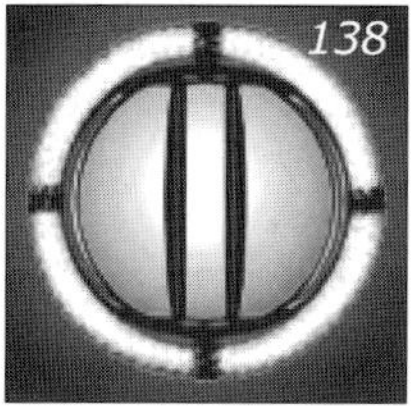

138

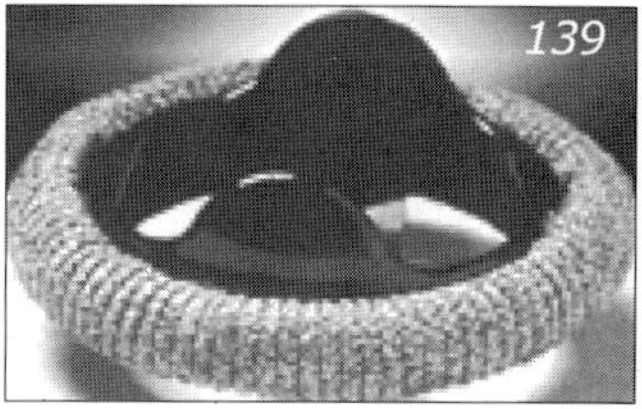

139

frequency of paravalvular leak. The St Jude Medical Regent aortic valve has an improved effective orifice area, achieved by reducing the sewing ring thicknes, shifting the carbon rim to the supra-annular position and improving the rotation mechanism *(Figure 140)*. Another model, called FlexCuff has a flanged and more pliable sewing ring that easily conforms to the annulus *(Figure 141)*.

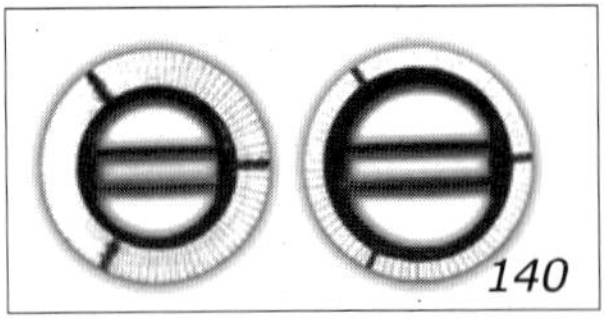

140

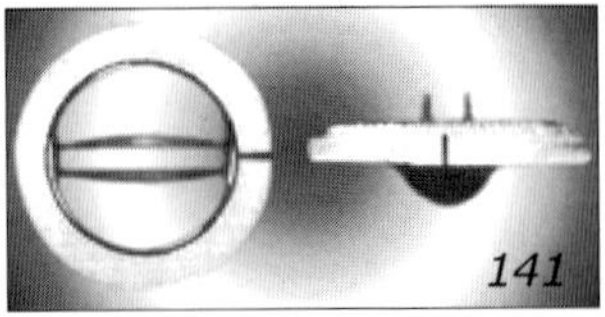

141

The CarboMedics (Sulzer CarboMedics, Inc., Austin, Texas) bileaflet prosthesis was introduced in 1986. It has a solid Pyrolite housing and flat leaflets of pyrolytic carbon coated over a tungsten–loaded graphite substrate. It has a radio–opaque titanium ring and increased tungsten content in the leaflet substrate. The opening angle of the leaflet is 78°. The leaflet pivot retention mechanism is within the housing without pivot guards, struts or orifice projections *(Figure 142)*. Leaflet motion is by rotation. The leaflets can be rotated within the housing. Apart from the standard models *(Figure 143)* several task–specific modified versions are available. The Carbo-Medics Top Hat *(Figure 144)* aortic

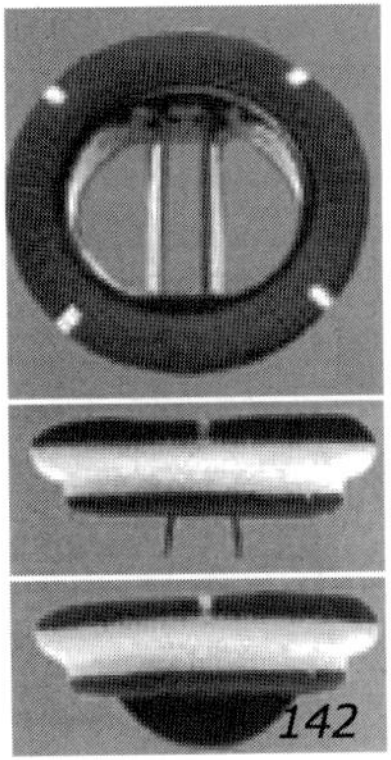

142

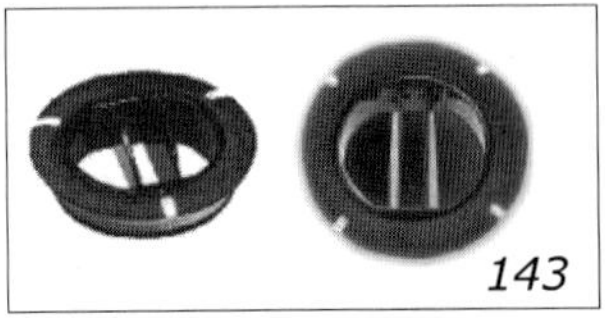

143

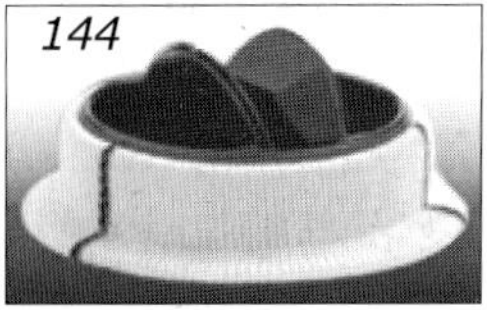

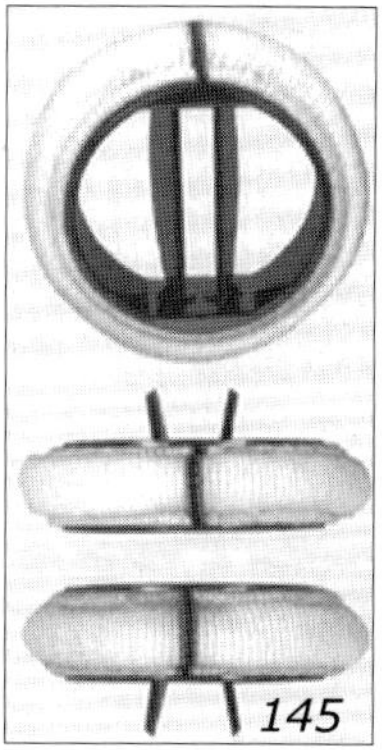

prosthesis is designed for supra-annular implantation and improved haemodynamic performance in small sizes. The Carbo- Medics Orbis Universal has a contoured sewing cuff *(Figure 145)* which facilitates its use for both mitral and aortic valve replacement. The SuMit design for mitral implantation reduces disc protrusion into the left ventricle *(Figure 146)*. The CarboMedics OptiForm Valve has a bulky but compliant sewing cuff *(Figure 147)* that can be optimally adapted to any problematic mitral annulus, particularly in difficult redo surgery or in the presence of heavy annular calcification. The Carbo-Medics Reduced Cuff Aortic Valve has a thinned out cork-shaped *(Figure 148)* sewing cuff which decreases the outside valve diameter without changing the internal orifice diameter. This facilitates the insertion of a relatively larger prosthesis. Paediatric-Small Adult valves are available in 16 and 18 mm sizes for both aortic and mitral positions. The balance between valve size and performance is expected to minimise patient-prosthesis mismatch and the consequent need for repeated valve replacements during the life of the child. The Sulzer Kinetic,

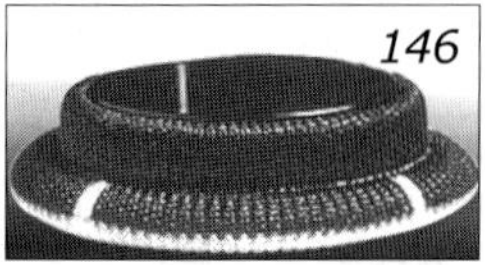

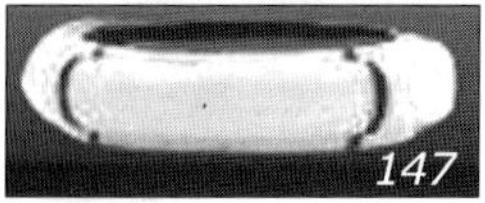

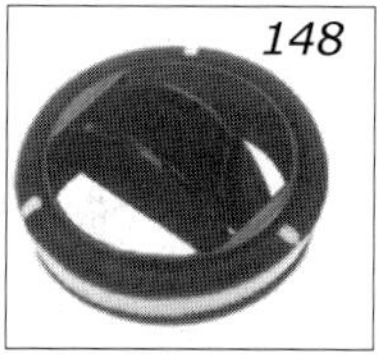

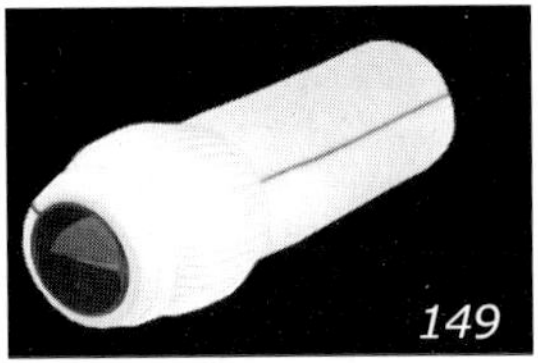

149

an evolving model, has valve size-related opening angles. This optimises the haemodynamic efficiency of the device.[113] An anatomically designed Carbo-Seal Valsalva ascending aortic prosthesis, which replicates the natural sinus, is now available *(Figure 149).*

150

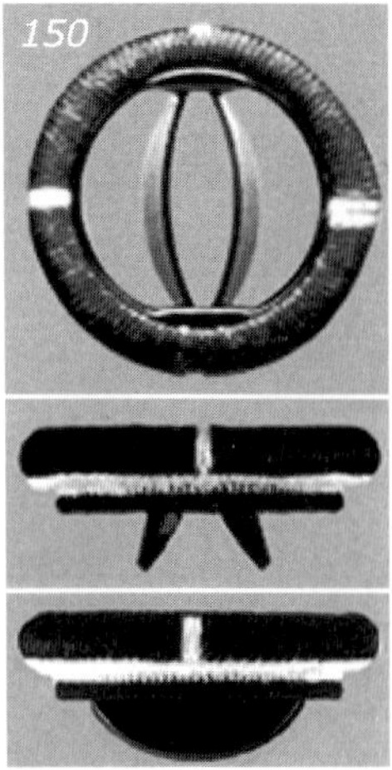

The Sorin Bicarbon (Sorin Biomedica, Saluggia, Italy) mechanical prosthesis is a rotatable bileaflet prosthesis with a titanium alloy housing coated with a thin film of pyrolytic carbon (Carbofilm), and curved leaflets with pyrolytic carbon coated over a graphite and tungsten substrate *(Figure 150)*. It has a titanium housing with aerofoil housing profile and a hinge mechanism that supports a rolling leaflet motion. The hinge cavity supports a constantly varying, single-point contact between pivot and housing. The opening angle of both the aortic and mitral prostheses is 70°. The sewing ring is made with Dacron and carbon-coated Teflon. Bicarbon valves are available in three configurations (Standard, Fitline and Slimline) for both the aortic and mitral models. The Standard aortic valve features a pliable cylindrical cuff designed

151

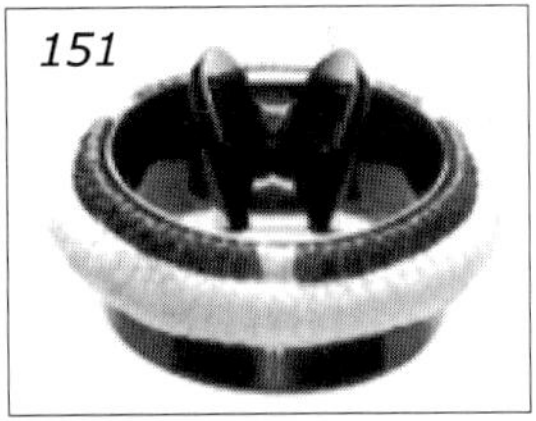

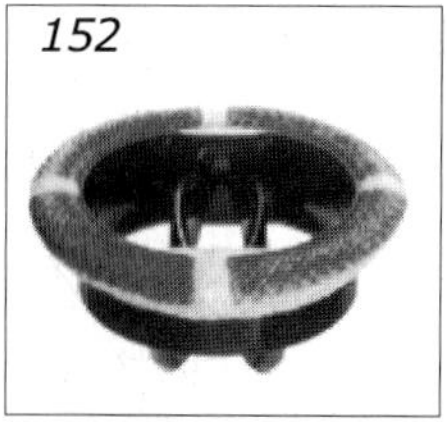

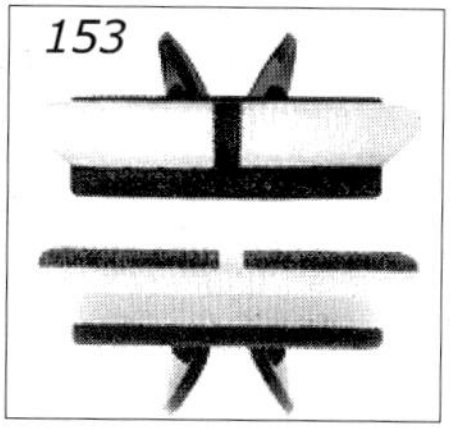

for supra-annular positioning *(Figure 151)* and the mitral valve features a large compliant cuff designed to conform to the irregularities of difficult annuli *(Figure 152)*. The Fitline *(Figure 153)* and Slimline *(Figure 154)* models incorporate cuff variations aimed at intra-annular and supra-annular placement, respectively, with an improved orifice–to–annulus ratio. Baxter acquired the rights to market the Sorin valve in the USA as the Edwards Mira valve, which is awaiting FDA approval. Mira has a modified sewing ring with a silicon sponge insert. This design, called StarRing, has been created by Albert Starr and is aimed at consonance with even the worst affected native annulus conditions. The unique hyperbolic shape of the mitral sewing ring provides a gradual curvature that increases the sealing surface area without compromising the orifice area *(Figure 155)*. The large sealing area permits a variety of suture techniques. This hyperbolic shape allows attachment to both atrial and ventricular sides for greater stability. The aortic sewing ring has a downstream extension which increases the zone of

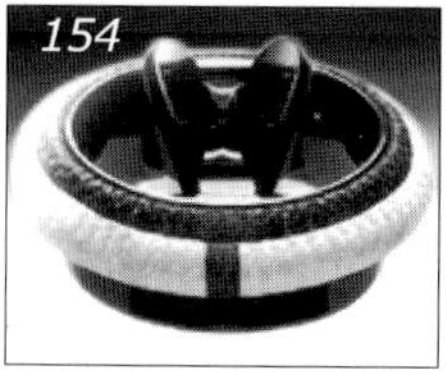

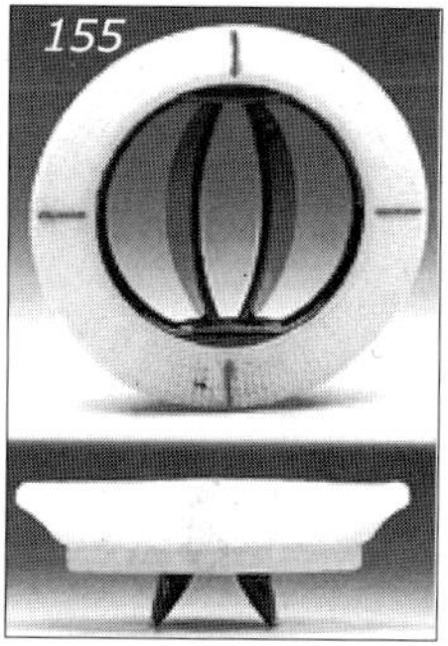

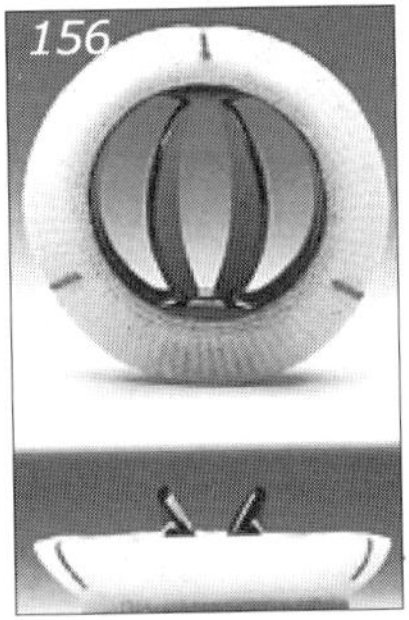

156

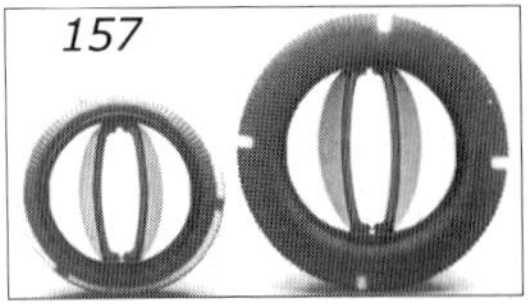

157

contact to improve valve seating *(Figure 156)*. Silicone sponge, like 'built-in' pledgets, allows sutures to be tied securely while supporting even the most delicate tissue. The counterpart of Sorin Slimline is known as the Mira Finesse valve.

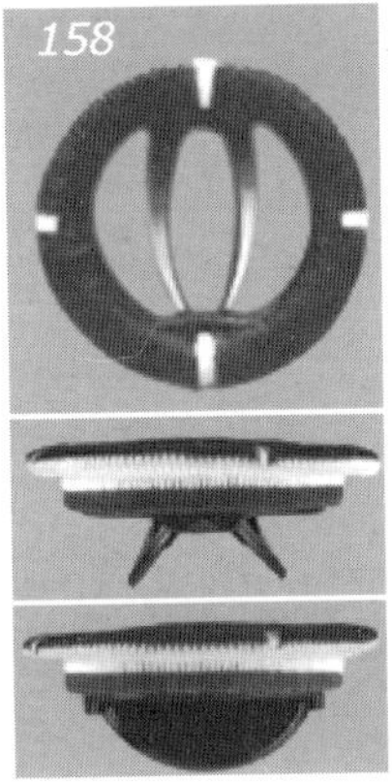

158

The Edwards Duromedics bileaflet valve *(Figure 157)* was originally designed and marketed by Hemex Scientific (first human implant:1982). The leaflets were curved and translated slightly in the direction of flow as they opened. They were seated on a ledge moulded into the housing. In the aortic and mitral models, the leaflets opened to 77° and 73° respectively. The pivot ball hinge closed by rotation and translation. Hemex was later taken over by Baxter Healthcare Corporation (Edwards CVS Division), Irvine, California; and Duromedics was marketed as Tekna after some design and manufacturing modifications *(Figure 158)*. It had a solid pyrolytic housing and curved leaflets with pyrolytic carbon coated over a tungsten-loaded graphite substrate. Housing stability was increased by a Stellite stiffener ring over a solid pyrolytic valve housing. The sewing ring had Dacron coated with Biolite carbon.

The ATS (Advancing the Standard) mechanical prosthesis (ATS Medical Inc., Minneapolis, Minnesota) is a bileaflet valve introduced in 1992. It has a pyrolytic carbon housing and pyrolytic carbon leaflets containing a graphite substrate *(Figure 159)*. Its principal design feature is a convex hinge mechanism with protrusions on the inner aspect of the housing that support the leaflets. There are no protruding struts with this hinge mechanism. The convex hinge mechanism is designed to facilitate retrograde washing. The valve is rotatable and has an opening angle of 85°. The Standard series valve *(Figure 160)* is intended for intra-annular placement whereas the Advanced Performance (AP) series, with a reduced cuff size *(Figure 161)*, is indicated for supra-annular placement where the tissue annulus is small but an optimal effective orifice area is desirable. The AP series valves are labelled in even numbers.

159

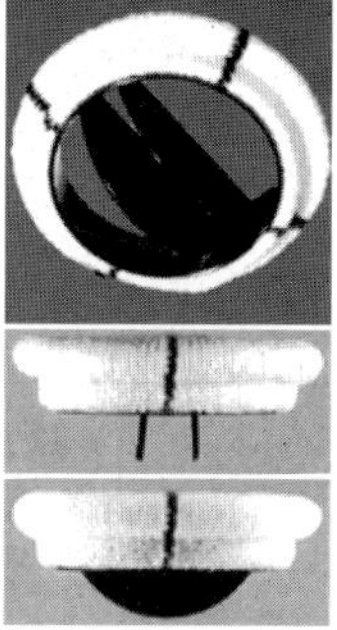

In 1994, Medtronic Incorporated, Minneapolis, Minnesota, began a clinical study on the Medtronic Parallel valve *(Figure 162)*, which was developed in cooperation with Carbon Implants, Inc. It was designed to open parallel to the flow with a 90° opening angle; to limit excessive regurgitation from a long closing arc, the closed angle was increased to 40°, which necessitated a

160

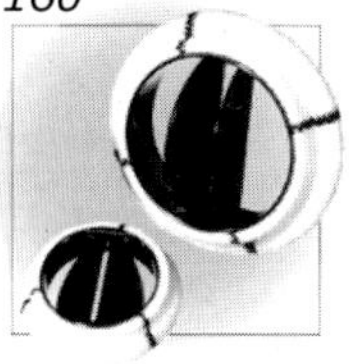

161

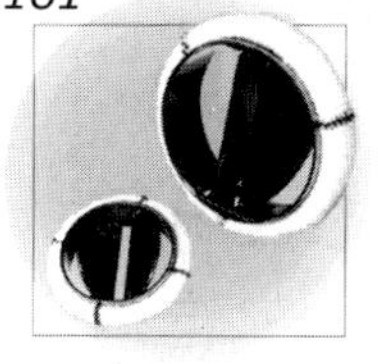

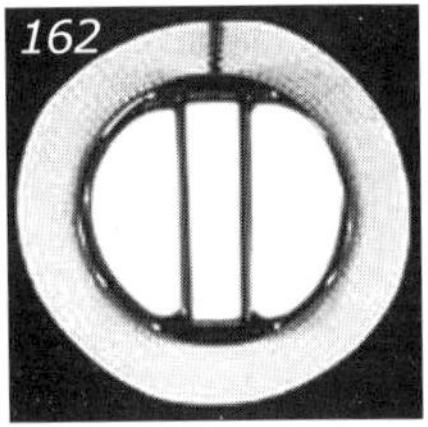

substantially longer orifice to contain the leaflets in the closed position. This design featured a relatively complex pivot with a feature intended to reduce leakage when the valve was fully closed. This pivot proved to be a notable risk factor for valvular thrombosis and the device was withdrawn shortly after the onset of clinical trials in Spain. The Advantage *(Figure 163)* pyrolytic carbon heart valve was another bileaflet valve put on trial by Medtronic. The first human implant in 1999 in Germany was followed by worldwide multicentric clinical trials. The valve features a large central flow opening designed to reduce velocity and blood turbulence. It has a pyrolytic carbon housing. The two pyrolytic carbon leaflets have an opening angle of 86 degrees. They close within the valve housing. Proprietary Sure–Flow "butterfly" pivot recesses are claimed to improve the process of washing the sensitive pivot regions, minimising the risk of thromboembolism.

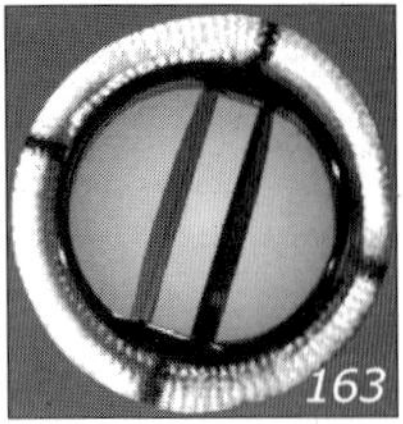

The Medical Carbon Research Institute, Austin, Texas introduced a pyrolitic carbon bileaflet prosthetic device called the On–X valve in 1996. It has a titanium–reinforced, rotatable Dacron sewing ring with carbon leaflets and housing. The aortic valve *(Figure 164)* features an elongated orifice with a flared inlet which improves flow and reduces pressure losses. The elongated orifice allows supra-annular positioning of the sewing ring so that

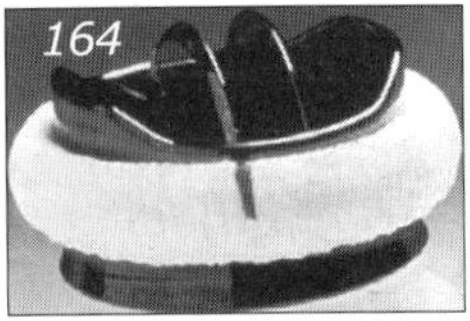

165

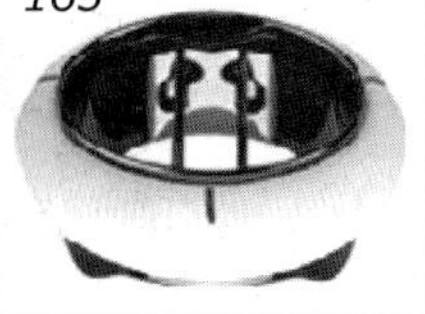

the thin flared inlet can be positioned in the annulus, interfacing directly with the aortic root. The elongated housing is claimed to reduce turbulence and lower transvalvular gradients. The mitral prosthesis *(Figure 165)* is also supra-annular with carbon leaflet guards positioned directly in the annulus to prevent impingement of the leaflet on the mitral apparatus. The On-X Conform bileaflet valve *(Figure 166)* with an extended sewing ring allows the device, as the name suggests, to conform to an irregular mitral valve annulus.

166

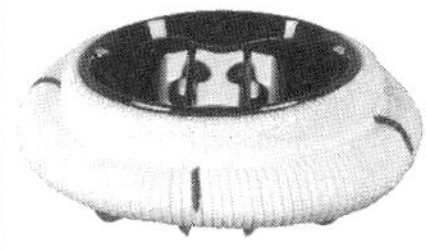

The Angelini 'Lamina-flo' bileaflet mechanical heart valve *(Figure 167)*, designed by Cardio Carbon Company Limited, Cheshire, UK features peripherally hinged leaflets which do not obstruct the blood flow on opening, greatly improving the valve hydrodynamics including reduced pressure drop. The device is fabricated from titanium alloy covered with a special diamond-like carbon coating for minimal wear and enhanced biocompatibility. The valve is under clinical trials.

The Jyros bileaflet heart valve was developed in the former Soviet Union in the mid-1980s, and became commercially available in the West in the early 1990s. Manufactured and distributed by Jyros Medical Devices (Jyros Worldwide Distrbution Ltd.), UK, the valve has an isotropic pyrolytic carbon housing and leaflets; a cobalt-chrome retaining ring

167

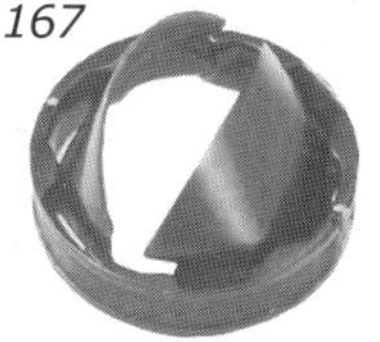

and a knitted polyester sewing ring *(Figure 168)*. The leaflets can rotate within the housing in response to the normal twisting flow pattern of the blood through the heart. The valve, labelled in even numbers, is fabricated in two size-related profiles: lower housing and higher housing.

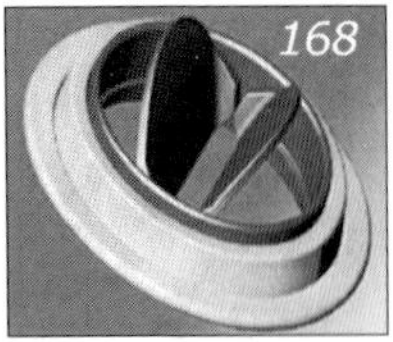

Medeng, an all-carbon bileaflet prosthesis *(Figure 169)* , is manufactured and distributed, probably within only limited areas, by Tecnology SRL of Argentina. TRI-Technologies of Nova Lima, Brazil had marketed a bileaflet prosthesis *(Figure 170)* with claims of unprecedented safety and optimised haemodynamic performance. However, recent reports of alleged device-related mortality in Italy and other countries have brought the device under investigators' scanner. Spain has ordered recall of the valve from the shelves.[114] In 1984, an Indian cardiac surgeon, Dr Dhani Ram Baruah and his wife Nirala Baruah, had designed a zirconium bileaflet valve coated with zirconium oxide, while they were in Glasgow, Scotland. A British patent (GB 2206182 A dated 29 December 1988) was sought for the device but the project was abandoned on account of Baruah's aversion to anticoagulants. Baruah later started his own Heart Valve Institute and Research Centre in Mumbai, India, to concentrate on tissue valves. A bileaflet design innovated by Kaster (US Patent 4488318 of 1984) had semiconical leaflets supported and constrained for pivotal movement between open

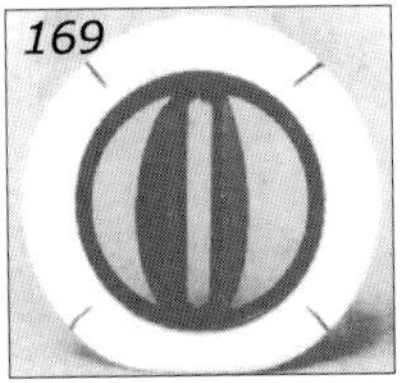

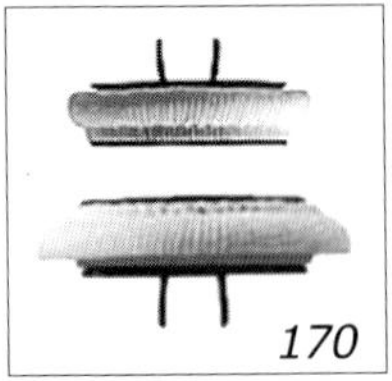

171

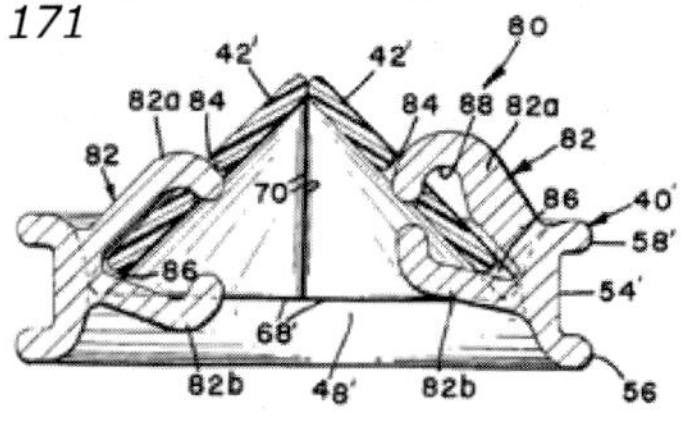

172

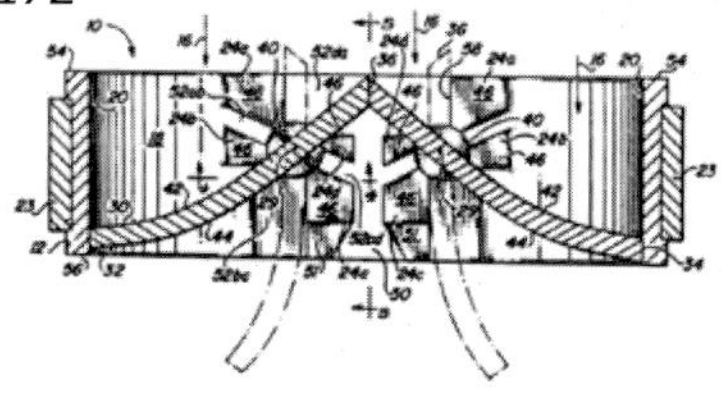

and closed positions by C–shaped arms engaging apertures and notches on the leaflets *(Figure 171)*. Carpentier proposed a bileaflet design (US Patent 4605408 of 1986) which has permanent magnets with opposing poles embedded in the leaflets and the orifice of the valve. The repelling force created by the opposing poles of the magnets is expected to modulate the leaflet movement. Dr Manuel Tascon along with Bokros had designed a bileaflet valve (US Patent 5080669 of 1992). The leaflets had pivotal enlargements and the valve body had spaced projections arranged in a fashion which would minimise stagnation in the region of the support arrangement *(Figure 172)*. Dr SHU Mark came up with a bileaflet valve design (International Patent 21305 of 1992) which had leaflets with composite curvature *(Figure 173)*. Dr Rainer H Frey of Starnberg, Germany had proposed a bileaflet valve (US Patent with 5607469 of 1997) with unequal leaflets *(Figure 174)*.

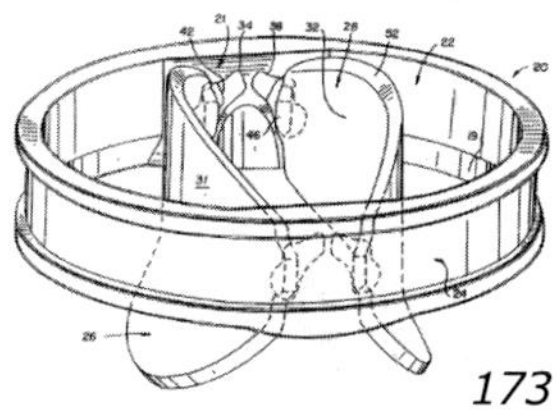

173

Tilting disc prostheses

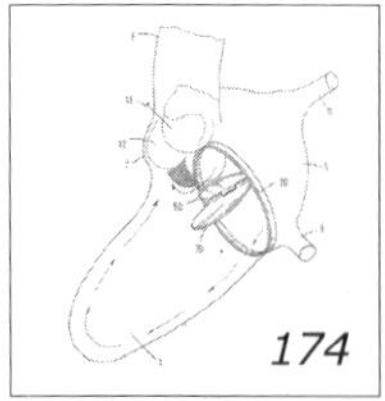

174

Björk had implanted a few Wada–Cutter valves at the Karolinska Institute in 1968 and was impressed by the basic design features and performance of this valve.[115] He persuaded Shiley to design and fabricate a more durable type of tilting disc prosthesis. As a result, the Björk–Shiley valve was designed and first implanted on 16 January 1969.[116,117] It became commercially available in 1971. The original model had a housing made from Haynes–25 alloy with two semihexagon-shaped metal struts which held a 'floating' Delrin disc in place *(Figure 175)*. The sewing ring was made from Teflon. After 1971, Delrin was replaced by pyrolitic carbon for durability and electronegativity. Initially it was a 'spherical' disc *(Figure 176)*. A radio-opaque marker ring was introduced in 1975. A year later the disc was redesigned and given a 'convexo-concave' shape. This must have been the first commercially available prosthetic valve with sewing ring configurations dedicated for intra-annular *(Figure 177)*, supra-annular *(Figure 178)* and subannular placement *(Figure 179)*. The aortic valve was available only for intra-annular implantation *(Figure 180)*.

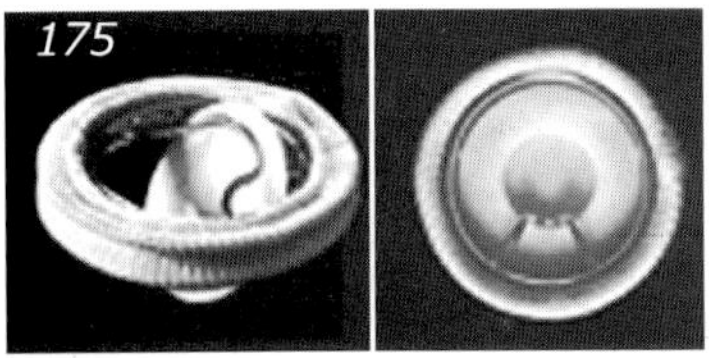

175

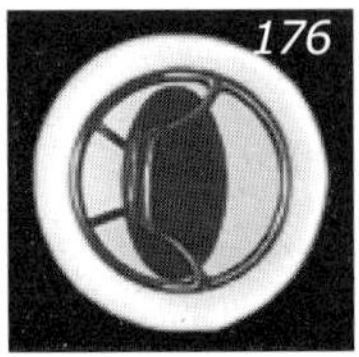

176

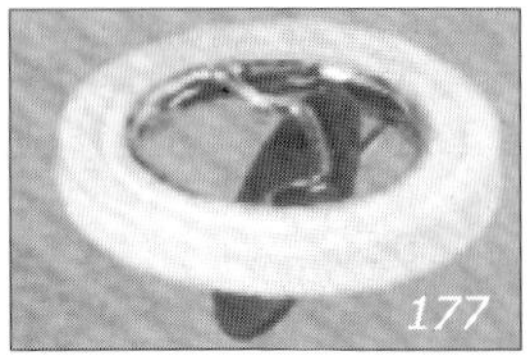

177

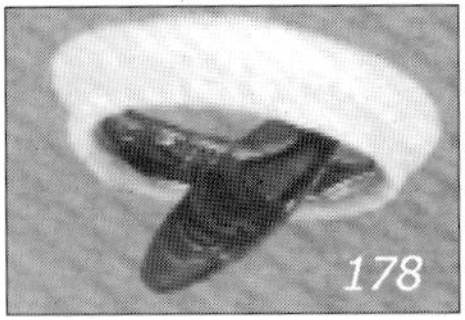

178

Unfortunately, these valves suffered an exceptionally high incidence of outflow strut fractures forcing discontinuance of the model within just five years. In 1981, the original strut on the outflow side was replaced by a single perpendicular strut and the product was christened Monostrut *(Figure 181)*. The orifice ring and integral struts are constructed from a single piece of cobalt–chromium alloy to give it a weld-free mechanism. A pyrolytic carbon disc contains a radiopaque tantalum marker. The opening angle is 70° and the valve can be rotated within the sewing ring. Leaflet motion is by rotation and translation. The aortic and mitral valves differ in their sewing ring configuration.The Björk–Shiley valve was initially manufactured and marketed by Shiley Laboratories, which was later purchased by Pfizer. Subsequently, the Monostrut valve was marketed by Sorin Biomedica, Saluggia, Italy and Alliance Medical Technologies, Inc., Irvine, California. The currently available model has a carbon-coated sewing ring *(Figure 182)*.

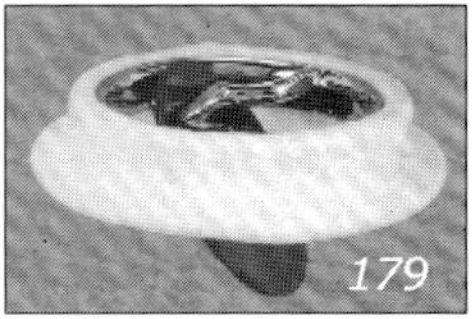

179

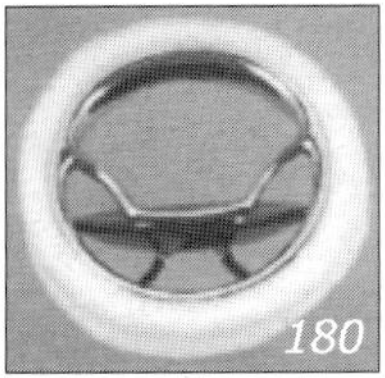

180

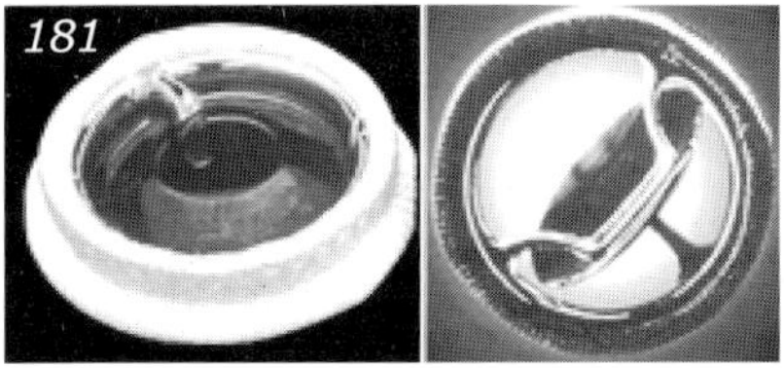

181

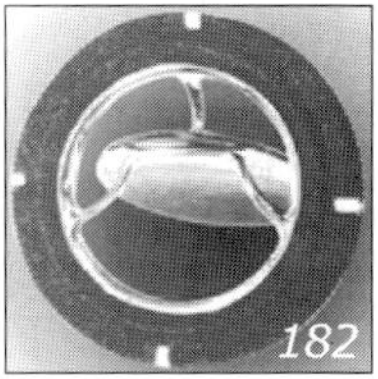

182

183

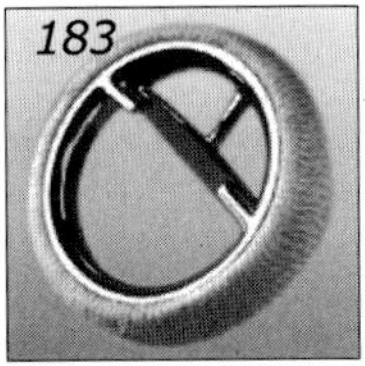

184

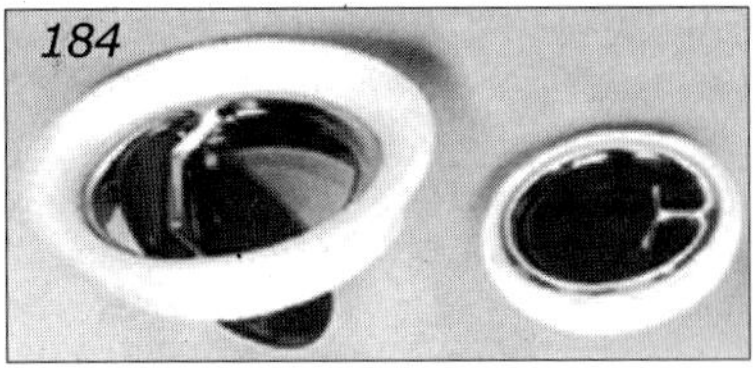

185

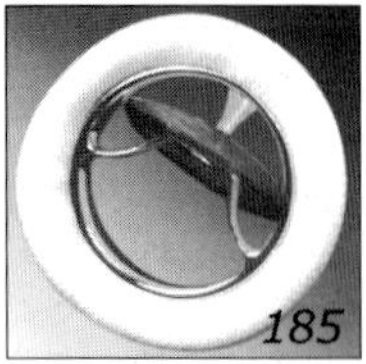

The basic design of the Monostrut valve was adopted by a few other tilting disc valves. The Bicer valve *(Figure 183)*, designed in 1984 by Dr Demetrio Bicer of Buenos Aires, Argentina had a pair of near-horizontal antithetically placed struts (US Patent 4494253 of 1985) to support the disc. The St Vincent, *(Figure 184)* valve, introduced in 1988 and marketed by Pacific Biomedical, Singapore had its single strut in the shape of a flattened Y. The Emiks valve *(Figure 185)*, designed in Russia, had a relocated main strut for unimpeded blood flow. The Indian-made TTK–Chitra valve *(Figure 186)*, distributed by TTK Pharma, Chennai, was subjected to extensive research and development[118] before its final acceptance for clinical use in 1989. The earliest model had a titanium housing with a welded strut and a Delrin disc. Subsequently, the housing and struts were integrally machined from a block of Haynes–25 coated with titanium nitride and the occluder was machined from a single crystal of synthetic sapphire. The final model has a Haynes–25 housing and a highly polished, cryo-machined solid-state disc manufactured from ultra high molecular weight polyethylene. The sewing ring is made from a knitted polyester fabric.

186

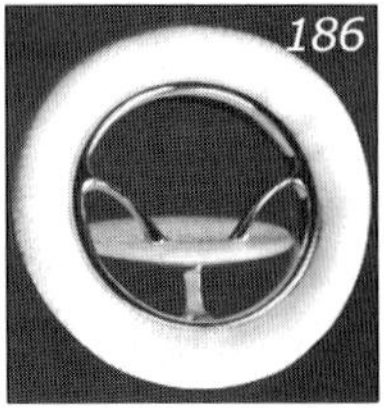

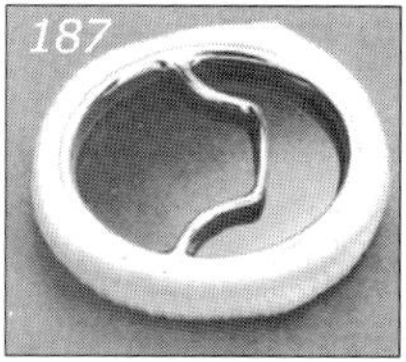

Sorin Biomedical, Saluggia, Italy manufactured a tilting disc valve patterned after the Björk–Shiley valve, but with both struts integral to the housing to avoid the possibility of strut fracture. The struts were contoured with a 'droplet' shaped cross-section, to facilitate better blood flow. The aortic and mitral sewing rings are configured in the same fashion as the Björk–Shiley valve. Monocast *(Figure 187)* , the first Sorin tilting disc valve, was implanted in 1977. This was modified to Carbocast *(Figure 188)*, introduced in 1986. It had a Carbofilm–coated cage. The currently available model is known as Allcarbon *(Figure 189)*. This monoleaflet mechanical prosthesis is constructed of a carbon–coated chromium alloy housing with a pyrolytic carbon disc. The sewing ring is also carbon coated.

The first modern–day pivoting disc prosthesis was the Lillehei–Kaster valve,[119] introduced in 1967 for both mitral and aortic positions *(Figure 190)*. It was a direct descendant of the Cruz–Kaster caged meniscus design. This valve had a weld-free titanium housing with diagonally opposite horn–like struts serving as disc retainers, a flat pyrolitic

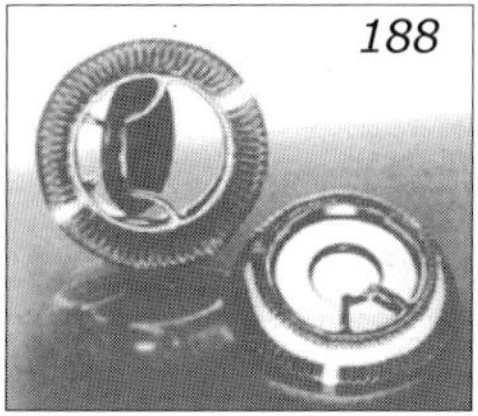

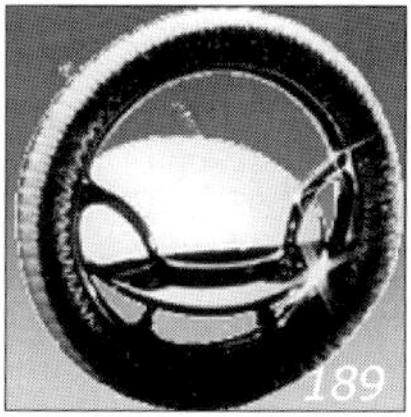

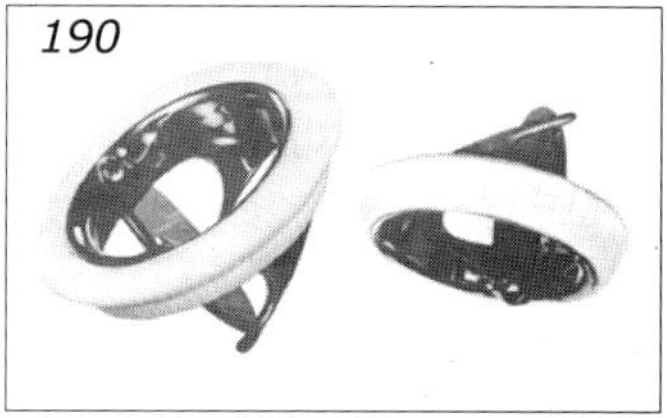

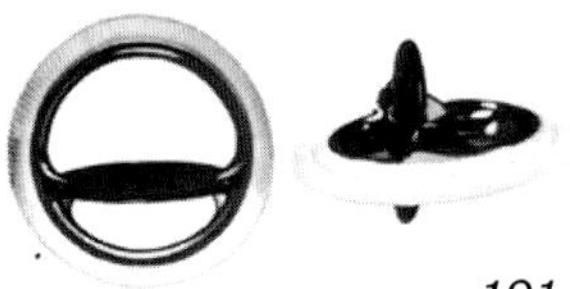

191

carbon–over–graphite disc and a seamless Teflon sewing ring. The long outflow struts and excursion of the disc into the ventricular chamber caused problems related to anatomical interference following mitral valve replacement.[120] This device was eventually modified, with considerably dwarfed struts and a concavoid disc, to be introduced as the Omniscience valve in 1976 (Medical Incorporated, Inver Grove Heights, Minnesota). The valve has an optimised pivot axis to allow central blood flow and a near-perpendicular opening angle *(Figure 191)*. In 1984, Omnicarbon, a modified version of the Omniscience valve, was introduced. Both the disc and housing are constructed from pyrolytic carbon *(Figure 192)*.

Dr Karl Victor Hall, of Rikshospitalet, a university hospital at Oslo, Norway, in the course of his practice faced the dilemma of choosing between two devices of almost balanced merit: the Björk–Shiley valve, designed by neighbourhood (Swedish) friend Björk and the Lillehei–Kaster valve, designed by a grandchild of son-of-the-soil Jens Kristian Lillehei who had left Norway in 1885 at the age of 17 to settle in the United States of America. These circumstances inspired Hall[121] to start a randomised study of the two valves. The outcome of this study prompted a hybrid configuration of the two valves. Hall teamed up with Kaster and a physicist–cum–businessman friend, Mr Arne Woien, to fabricate the Hall–

192

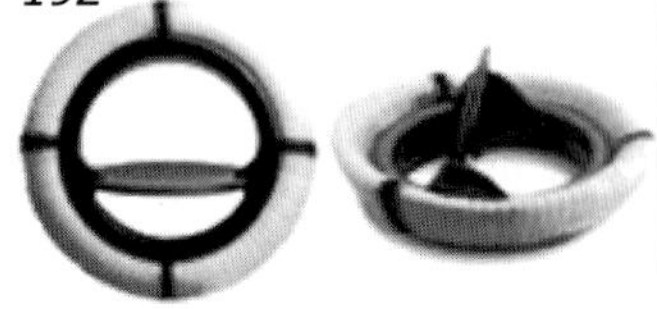

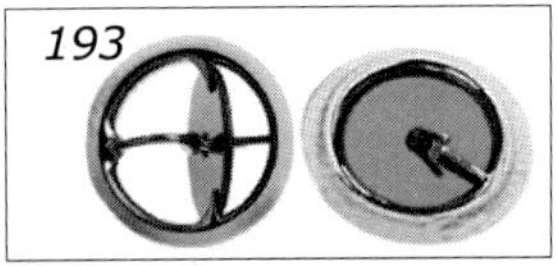

Kaster valve. They introduced a design modification that replaced the outflow struts with a central wire guide running through the disc. This valve was eventually sold to Medtronic and commercially launched as the Medtronic–Hall valve in 1977. The housing and central guide are made of titanium and the disc consists of pyrolytic carbon with a tungsten–loaded substrate for radiopacity. The disc has a single hole in its centre. This hole is used to mount the disc on a single, goose–neck shaped central strut, and the disc rides up and down on the strut. A second, smaller strut stops the motion of the disc when fully open *(Figure 193)*. Apart from the usual sizes in aortic and mitral models, the Medtronic–Hall aortic valve is also sold labelled as 20, 22 and 24 mm, respectively, wherein the sewing rings of larger sizes have been debulked to facilitate improved haemodynamics. The Medtronic–Hall Easy–Fit valve *(Figure 194)* features a new split–ring sewing cuff design intended only for supra-annular placement. It is expected to provide a greater orifice diameter-to-tissue annulus ratio.

Two European tilting disc valves, Liks–2 (Jyros Medical) and Ultracor (AorTech International, Strathclyde, Scotland), were introduced in 1982 and 1983, respectively. The former, designed and predominantly used in the erstwhile Soviet Union, has a curved disc with a depressed centre which hitches against a strut in the shape of a curly bracket *(Figure 195)*. The Ultracor

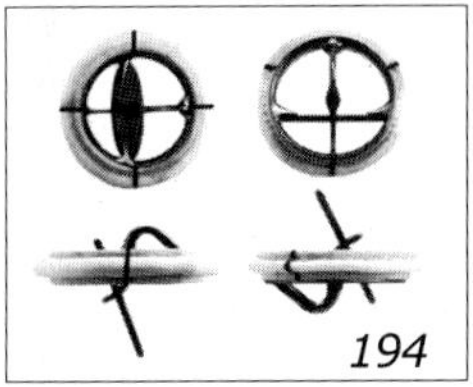

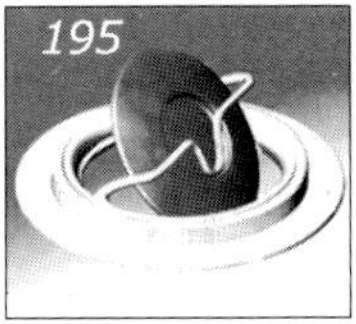

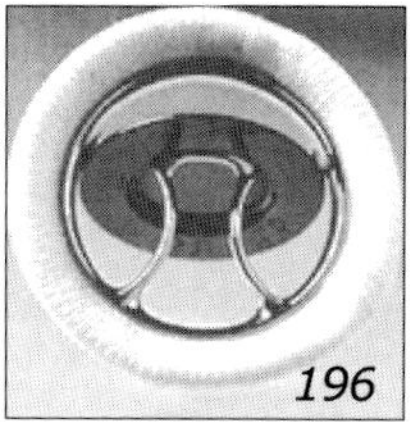
196

valve *(Figure 196)* is the third (after the Lillehei–Kaster and Hall–Kaster) tilting disc valve designed by Kaster. It has a plano–convex disc with pyrolytic carbon coating on a tungsten–impregnated graphite core. The aortic prosthesis has a 73° opening angle whereas the mitral prosthesis has a 68° opening angle. The housing is machined from a single block of titanium. It is popular in Great Britain and several other European countries. Another Russian valve called Planics *(Figure 197)* has similar features but to an extent resembles the Omniscience valve. Helmut Reul and associates[122] from the Helmholtz Institute for Biomedical Engineering, Aachen, Germany have introduced a new concept of single leaflet mechanical prosthesis in which pins by the side of the leaflets are guided into oblong bore-holes in the housing *(Figure 198)*. This is claimed to provide an automatic self cleansing effect.

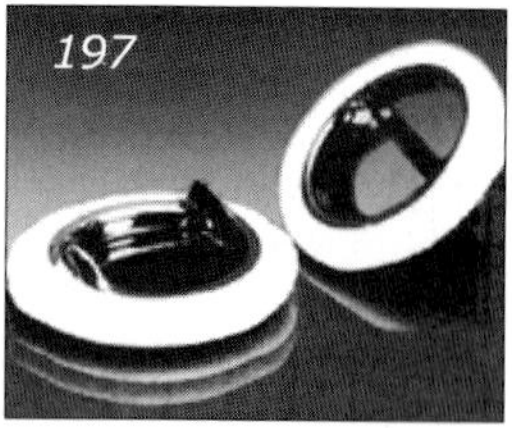
197

The Chinese manufactured Beijing GK heart valve prosthesis was designed by the Fuwai Cardiovascular Disease Hospital, Chinese Academy of Medical Sciences. This is the first hook–hole pivotal disc valve to receive a Chinese patent. It came into clinical use in 1985 and a second generation design, known as Beijing GK–2, is now available *(Figure 199)*. The other variety of

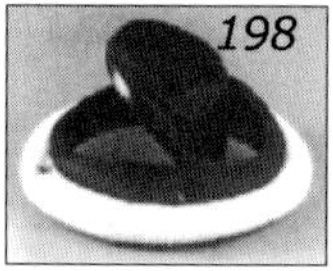
198

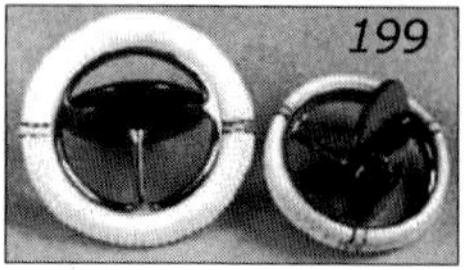
199

200

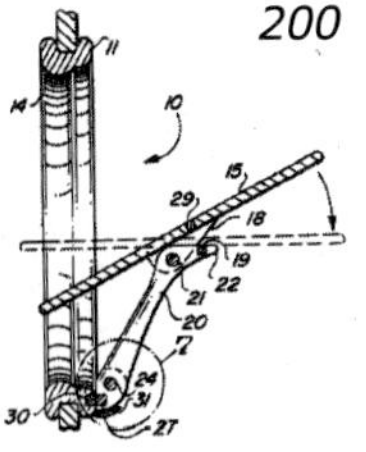

Chinese mechanical prosthesis, the Shanghai valve, has designs which appear to be clones of Bjork-Shiley, Monostrut, Bicer and other allied valves.

Dr Henry S Zibelin had conceptualised a single leaflet valve with a link bracket attached to one side of the disc and the valve housing with a movable link bridging the two (US Patent 4657545 of 1987). The mechanism was supposed to function with the help of two attracting permanent magnets positioned at the base of the link and valve ring; and two repelling magnets placed on the disc and its link system *(Figure 200)*. A group of German physicians and biomedical engineers led by Dr Hanns Pietsch described a solitary disc which was hinged to the housing by a flat, flexible lug inserted through a slot (US Patent 4643732 of 1987). Another group from the Federal republic of Germany comprising Dr Marti Knoch and others blueprinted the concept (US Patent 4775378 of 1988) of deploying an S-shaped occluder *(Figure 201)* expecting improved overall performance.

Biological heart valves

201

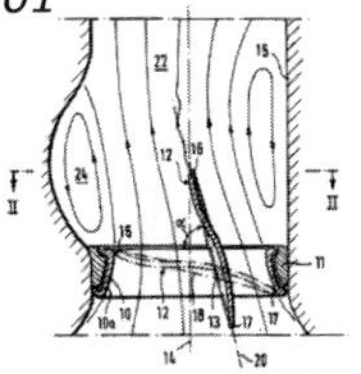

Bioprosthetic heart valves currently available or under development are classified in terms of tissue type, design and tissue treatment.[123] Tissue types include pericardial tissue and native valves. These materials are generally derived from bovine, porcine or human sources. The majority of contemporary biological valvular prostheses are constructed from bovine pericardium or porcine aortic valves. They are available in either stented or stentless varieties. Bovine pericardial prostheses use pressure-free fixation with glutaraldehyde which cross–links collagen and, at fixation pressures approaching zero, the collagen crimp framework is maintained to varying degrees. The natural aortic valve possesses unique architectural and material characteristics consonant with physiological function. Tissue preservation methods and stent designs define the anatomical characteristics and biomechanical properties of the leaflets. Initially introduced (first–generation) porcine bioprostheses had the tissue fixed with glutaraldehyde at high pressure (60–80 mmHg). Current–generation porcine prostheses use either low pressure or zero pressure glutaraldehyde fixation technology.

The prima facie role of glutaraldehyde in the calcification and subsequent mechanical degradation of bioprosthetic material has generated considerable concern in recent years. Various pre- and post-glutaraldehyde tissue treatment measures have been investigated in an attempt to offset these effects. They include chondroitin sulphate, sodium dodecyl sulphate, protamine, heparin, diphosphonates, glutamic acid, amino acids, lipid extraction, alpha–amino oleic acid, homocysteic acid, trivalent metal ions, ethanol, long chain alcohols, toluidine blue and various other detoxification methods. The last word on antimineralisation research is yet to be spoken. Fierce competition in this area has forced valve manufacturers to use proprietary nomenclature without divulging the exact nature of the calcium mitigation agent used.

Other steps in this direction include a thorough prepackaging rinse for the product to wash away free aldehydes followed by package in saline and gamma–irradiation. Preservation agents other than aldehydes are being enthusiastically tried out. Research is underway with alternative collagen cross-linking substances that include incorporative agents like epoxides in various combinations or hexamethylene di-isocyanate, and nonincorporative agents like acyle azide, carboliimide or dye-mediated photo-oxidation. Chemical modifications with various other agents such as polyglycidal ethers, cyanimide, glycerol, genipin and disuccinimidyl glutarate are also being undertaken. [123,124]

To a limited extent, autologous human pericardial tissue and native human heart valves have also been used as source material for tissue valves. They involve potentially lower immunogenic response, especially when native allograft and autograft valves have been used. These are used as non-stabilised material, and include homografts as well as cryopreserved cadaver allografts. More recently, decellularized and non–fixed human or porcine valves have been implanted clinically.

Stented pericardial valves

The disappointing experience with the earlier pericardial prostheses prompted further research aimed at analysing the causes of their failure. Edwards Laboratories took the lead in trying out various modifications in this direction.[125] Experimental trials with the Edwards pericardial xenografts began in 1976. Carpentier associated himself with the project in 1979, and the first human implantation of a Carpentier–Edwards bovine pericardial aortic valve took place in 1980. Vascor Incorporated,[126] Anaheim, California presented a stented pericardial valve *(Figure 202)* in 1981. The aortic model had a scalloped inflow configuration and a semiflexible orifice. The undulating sewing ring followed the anatomy of the normal annulus. By contrast the mitral valve had a flat and rigid inlet which was contoured to provide a smoother flow transition from the atrium to the ventricle. Dr Shlomo Gabbay of the Albert Einstein College of Medicine, Bronx, New York, presented a unicusp concept of stent-mounted bovine pericardial xenograft at the annual meeting of the Society of Thoracic Surgeons held in 1984.[127] Manufactured by Meadox Medical, the valve had a glutaraldehyde-fixed single pericardial leaflet mounted on a flexible Delrin stent covered with pericardium *(Figure 203)*. Both these valves were probably put to only limited human use.

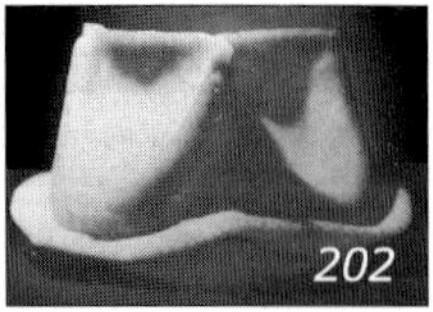

202

After initial hiccups, the concept of bovine pericardium seems to have been rescued as an acceptable alternative for valve fabrication by the Carpentier-Edwards valve, which established itself as a leading contemporary stented pericardial xenograft. Each of its three leaflets is carved by a computer-aided technique for stress-free leaflet-to-stent matching. Leaflets achieve satisfactory coaptation without stent post sutures. The tissue is mounted on a lightweight Elgiloy frame that is covered with knitted polytetrafluoroethylene fabric. Initially it was designed only for the aortic position. Subsequently, the Carpentier-Edwards bovine pericardial mitral valve was available for human use. Currently, two aortic models are available, the Carpentier-Edwards Perimount (Model 2700) pericardial

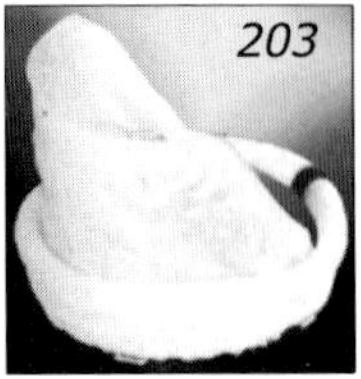

203

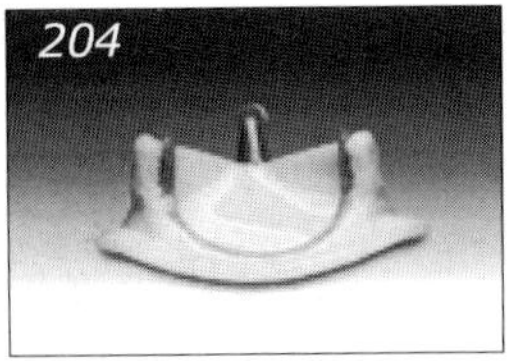

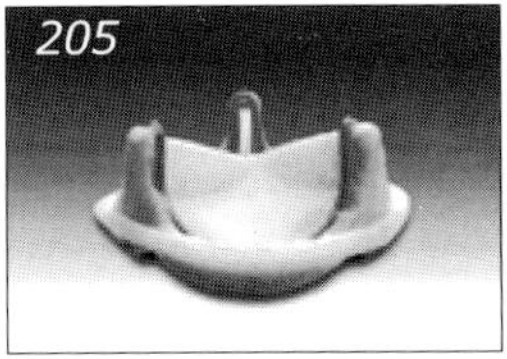

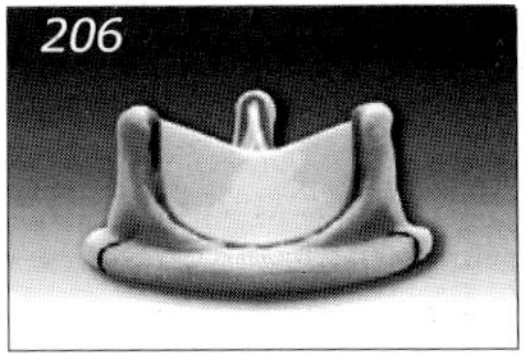

bioprosthesis *(Figure 204)* and the Carpentier–Edwards Perimount RSR (reduced sewing ring: Model 2800) pericardial bioprosthesis *(Figure 205*). The Carpentier–Edwards Perimount–Plus (Model 6900P) pericardial bioprosthesis is designed for the mitral position *(Figure 206)*. It is claimed that these models incorporate optimum material choice for both tissue and stent; integrated processes such as Neutralogic stress-free fixation, PeriMap pericardial thickness mapping technology, and tissue deflection testing enable the leaflets to be accurately matched. Anticalcific treatment with XenoLogiX is expected to enhance the longevity of the device.

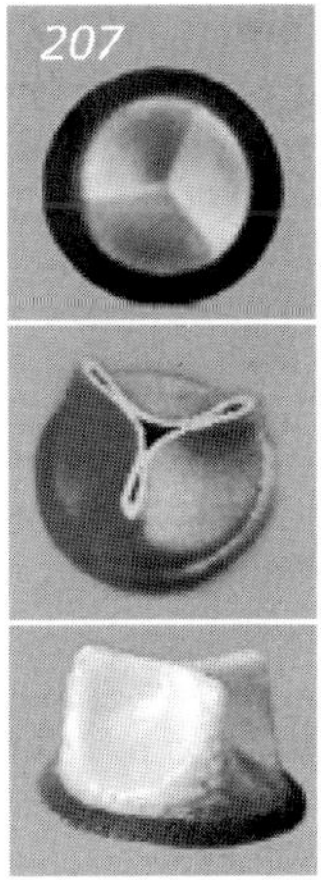

The Mitroflow pericardial bioprosthesis (Mitroflow International Inc., Richmond, British Columbia, Canada), now available as Synergy PC (Sulzer CarboMedics) is made with a Delrin stent for flexibility and pericardium fixed at zero-pressure with glutaraldehyde. The treated pericardium is utilised as a single component without critical stent–post sutures *(Figure 207)*.

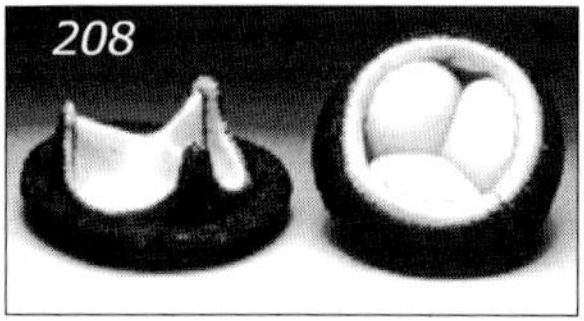

The Sorin Pericarbon More pericardial bioprosthesis is made with two sheets of pressure-free fixed pericardium over a

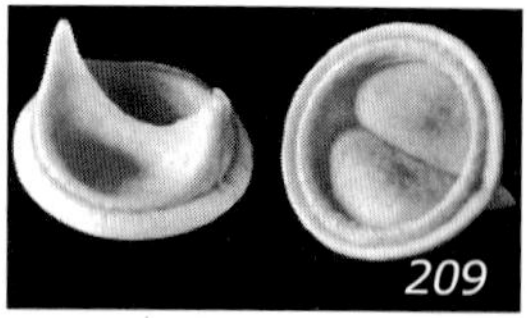

Delrin stent. One sheet forms three cusps with zero stress on the commissures and a cylindrical shape in the open position. The other sheet coats the inner surface of the stent. The prosthesis is low profile, has a radiopaque metal wire marker and a Carbofilm (a proprietary carbostatic carbon) coated Dacron fabric in the sewing ring *(Figure 208)*.

Baruah designed bovine pericardial xenografts in 1986. Initially, they were mounted on a cloth-covered rigid stent, which was later replaced by a pericardium-covered, flexible, high-density polymer stent. The Baruah mitral valves were manufactured in bileaflet *(Figure 209)* and trileaflet *(Figure 210)* configurations. The ultra-low profile tricuspid valves were manufactured in a trileaflet configuration *(Figure 211)*. The valve was conceived as an anatomical facsimile with one large anterior leaflet and smaller posterior and septal leaflets. Baruah did not offer any stented valve for the aortic position. Marketed by Medos Medizintechnik of Germany, these valves were first implanted clinically around 1990 in a

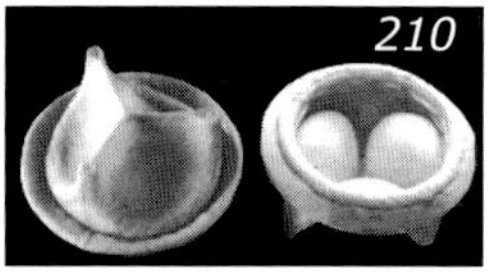

few hospitals in India and the Prince of Wales Hospital in Hong Kong. With the introduction of Baruah stentless

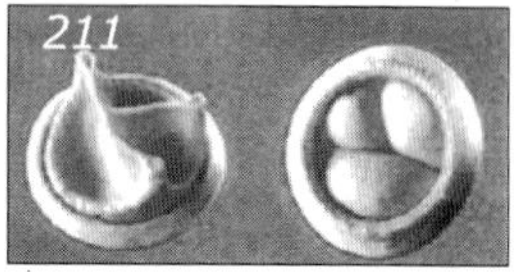

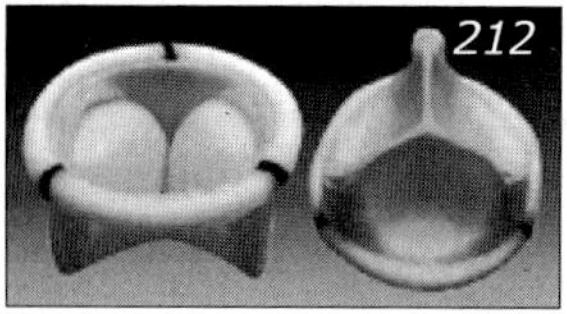

212

pericardial valves, interest in the stented variety gradually diminished. The Braile BioproPB stented

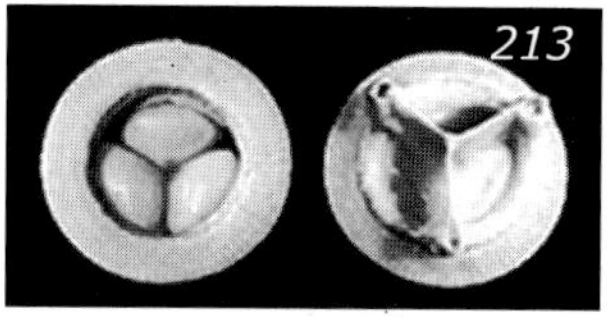

213

bovine pericardial bioprosthesis *(Figure 212)*, designed in 1977 by Dr DM Braile of the Instituto de Molestias Cardiovasculares, Sao Jose do Rio Preto, Brazil and marketed by Braile Biomedicas Inc., is mounted on a Delrin support with the three shafts also coated with pericardium. This bioprosthesis is also marketed as Macchi valve. Biomed *(Figure 213)* and Fisics–Incor *(Figure 214)*, are two other stented pericardial valves from South America, developed by Biomedica Mexicana and the Heart Institute of Sao Paolo, Brazil, respectively. In China, unnamed locally made pericardial prostheses *(Figure 215)* have also been put to use.

The CarboMedics Photofix Alpha is a bovine pericardial stented bioprosthesis *(Figure 216)* in which dye–mediated photo-oxidation relies on methylene blue and light to create new cross-links in collagenous

214

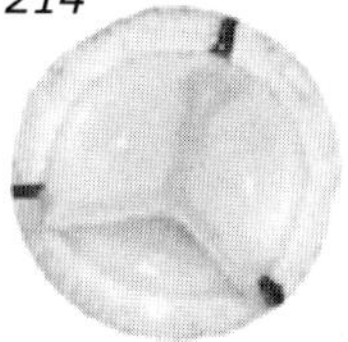

215

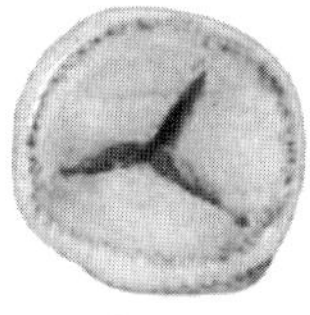

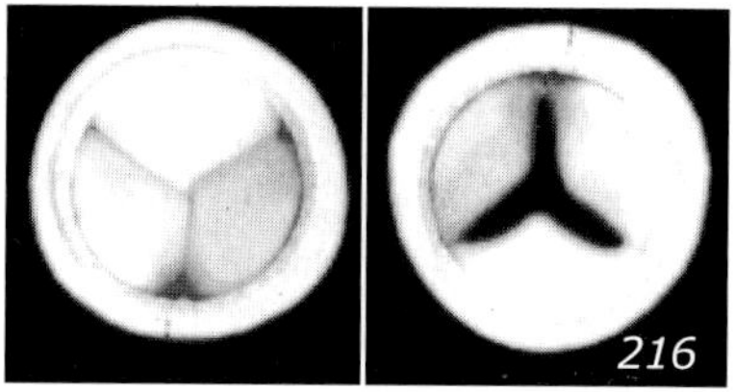

216

substrate material without the use of aldehydes. The tissue is placed in a phosphate-buffered saline solution containing the photoactive methylene blue dye, and light of an appropriate wave length is used to activate the dye catalyst. This highly reactive oxygen free radical interracts in turn with specific collagen amino acid side chains to form new cross-links. Bio Medical Design, Inc, Atlanta, Georgia have developed a carboliimide cross-linked porcine valve *(Figure 217)* for experimental and subsequent clinical trials.

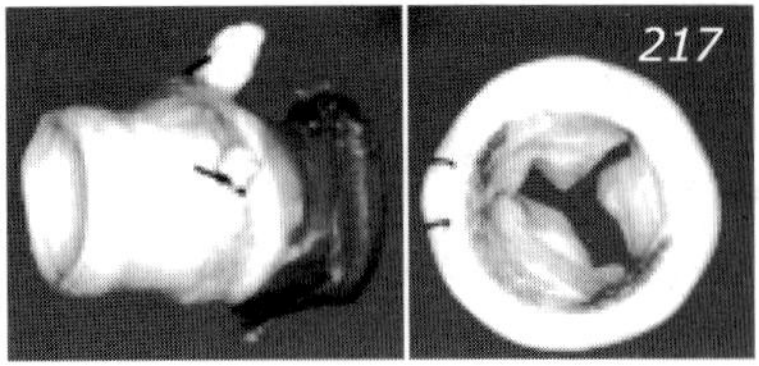
217

Dr Jack W Love of Santa Barbara, California patented the unique concept (US Patent 4470157 of 1984) of a prefabricated kit comprising two stents and a sewing ring, capable of instant valve assembly. This was further refined as a 'Rapid assembly, concentric mating stent tissue heart valve with enhanced clamping and tissue alignment' and patented (US Patent 5163955 of 1992). This innovative valve concept has recently been commercialised by Autogenics, Newbury Park, California. It allows the surgeon to fabricate a heart valve made out of the patients own pericardium during surgery. The Autogenics kit consists of tools *(Figure 218)* to create the valve in a matter of minutes: a cookie-cutter type tool for obtaining the

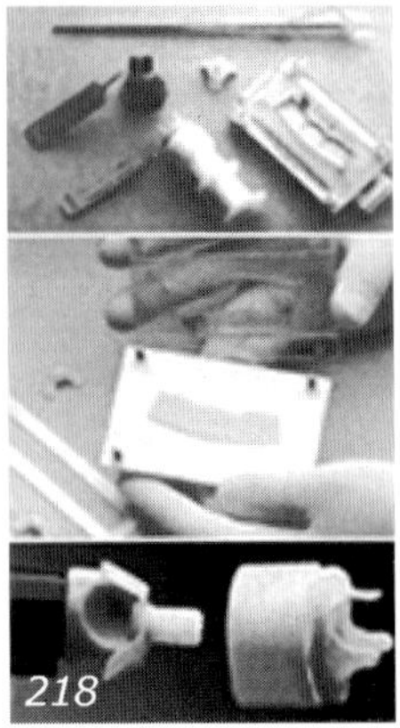
218

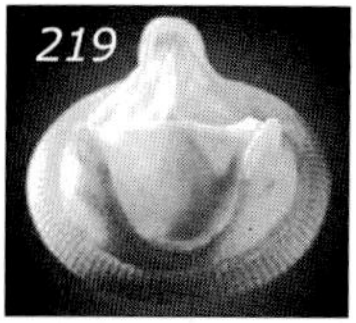

correctly shaped piece of pericardium, a frame that snaps together around the tissue, and a holder to precisely align two pieces for assembly. A piece of the

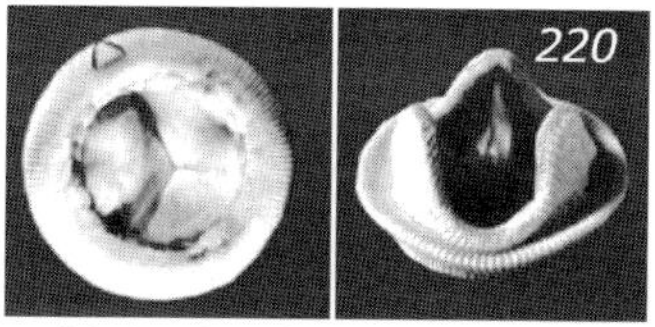

patient's pericardium is briefly fixed in glutaraldehyde solution to stiffen and stabilise it; then it is cut using the template. This results in a strip of tissue to form the three valve cusps. This tissue is wrapped around the inner frame, and is then wedged between the inner and outer stents to hold it in place. The completed valve *(Figure 219)* is inspected for any leak, and implanted in the usual manner.

Stented porcine valves

The Hancock Standard porcine valve *(Figure 220)* by Medtronic was the first commercially available stented porcine valve. It had a flexible polypropylene stent with a radiopaque ring of cobalt–chromium alloy added for rigidity. On account of the right coronary cusp muscular shelf, which compromised the valve's haemodynamic efficiency, this valve made way for the 'modified orifice' composite design porcine valve *(Figure 221)*. Once the offending right coronary cusp with its flow–impeding muscle shelf was replaced with a non-coronary cusp from another valve, the three flexible leaflets opened completely and symmetrically to offer minimal obstruction to blood flow. It used high

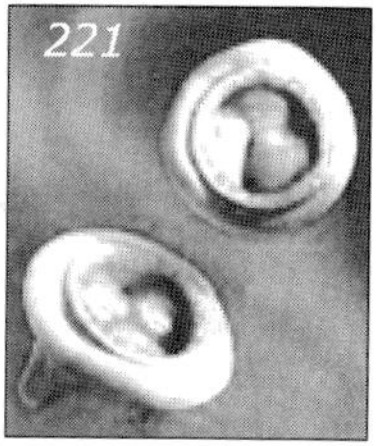

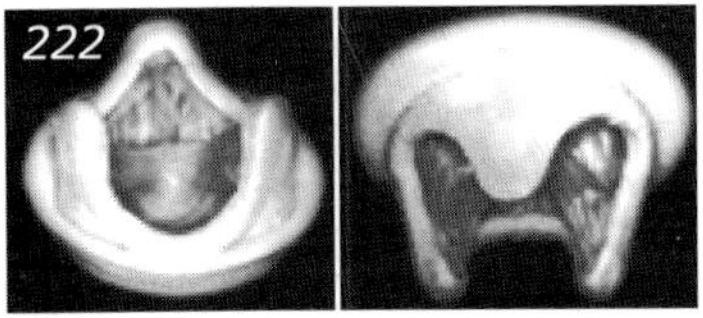

pressure fixation technology without any tissue treatment. The Hancock II valve *(Figure 222)* incorporates second-generation

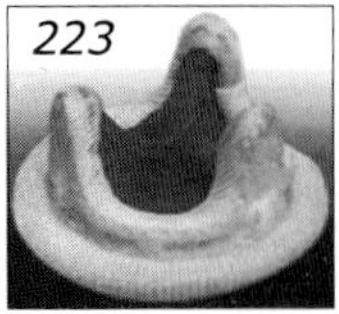

features such as low-pressure fixation, calcification retardant treatment, a thinner stent and a modified scalloped aortic sewing ring for supra-annular placement. The Medtronic Intact valve *(Figure 223)* has a distinctive blue colour on account of its calcification-retardant treatment with toluidine blue. It is fixed at zero-pressure rendering the leaflets thinner and more pliable. Medtronic have recently introduced their third-generation Mosaic valve with Cinch implant system for ease of insertion *(Figure 224)*. It is subjected to what is described as 'physiologic fixation' wherein the tissue is fixed with glutaraldehyde at zero-pressure and the aortic wall is predilated to reduce deformation of the commissures. The prosthesis is treated with alpha amino oleic acid to retard calcification. This prosthesis allows for true supra-annular placement with the sewing ring flush with the inflow edge of the stent (Supra-X positioning).

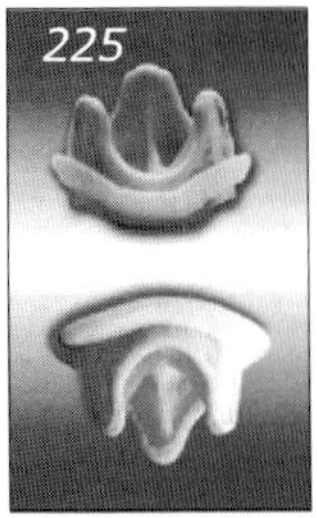

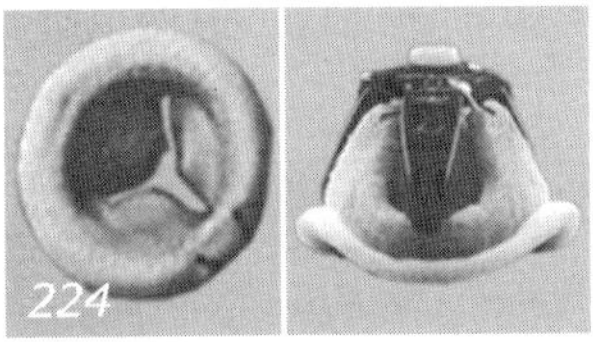

Baxter's Carpentier-Edwards standard porcine valve *(Figure 225)* became available shortly after the Hancock valve. The frame of the valve is a flexible wire

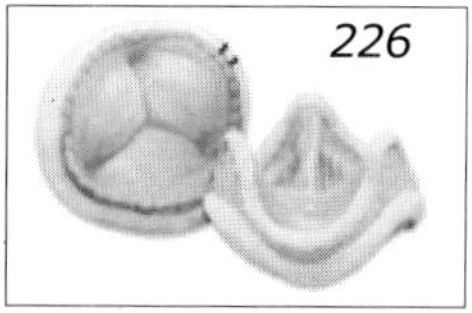

226

stent intended to reduce stress on the leaflets and orifice while retaining its original contour over time. A one-piece, cylindrical, flexible Mylar support surrounds a flexible wire frame. The annulus is asymmetrical rather than circular to incorporate the muscular septal ridge of the porcine right coronary cusp. Changing with the times, the Carpentier–Edwards standard valve is now processed by low-pressure fixation instead of the original high-pressure fixation. In the Carpentier–Edwards Supra-annular porcine bioprosthesis *(Figure 226)*, the mounting structure of the aortic valve has been redesigned for positioning above the annulus.The fixation treatment and the stent have been modified in an attempt to improve leaflet durability. The sewing ring was reconfigured to increase the effective orifice of the valve. The prosthesis has a reduced stent profile and the tissue, preserved with glutaraldehyde at low fixation pressure, is treated with polysorbate 80. Carpentier–Edwards Duralex *(Figure 227)*, a mitral valve bioprosthesis with an extended suture ring for better annular adaptation is also currently available.

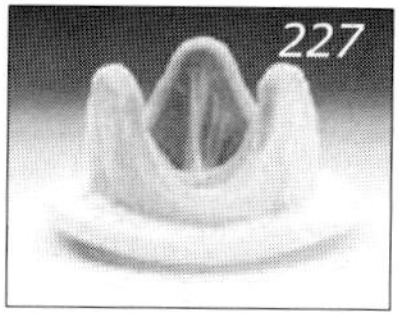

227

The original low-profile Liotta porcine bioprosthetic valve was manufactured by Biocor Industria e Pesquisa Ltda, Brazil. For some time it was sold as the Biocor–Genetic valve (marketed by Genetic Laboratories, Inc) and also as the St Jude BioImplant valve. It is now available internationally as the St Jude Medical Biocor valve, a zero-pressure glutaraldehyde-fixed device manufactured from individually selected triple–composite porcine aortic valve leaflets devoid of a septal muscle

228

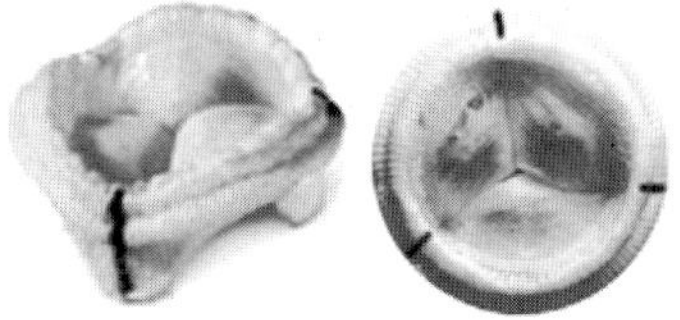

229

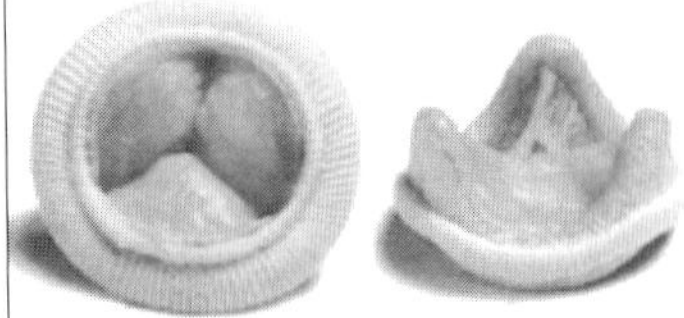

bar *(Figure 228).* Recently St Jude Medical have introduced Epic, a modified version of the Biocor valve which incorporates a proprietary anticalcification technology called Linx. Synergy ST (Sulzer CarboMedics), originally Labcor (Labcor Laboratories Ltda, Brazil), is another stented porcine valve *(Figure 229)* with a tricomposite design.

Other contemporary stented porcine valves include Tissuemed or Aspire valve *(Figure 230)*, originally designed by the cardiac research unit of Killingbeck Hospital, Leeds, manufactured by Tissuemed Ltd, Leeds, and now marketed by Aortech International, Scotland; Braile Biopro PP *(Figure 231)* from Braile Biomedicas; Biomed *(Figure 232)* manufactured

230

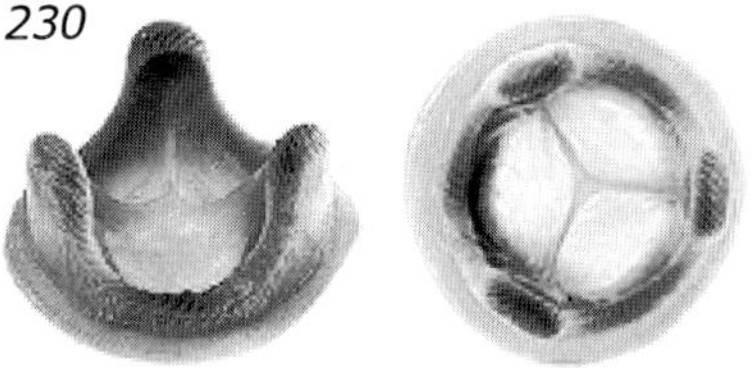

231

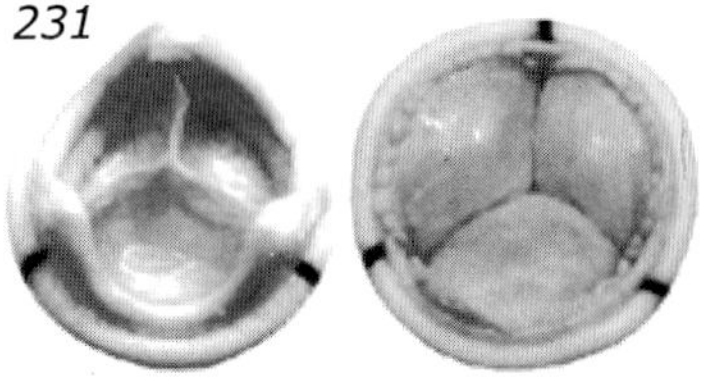

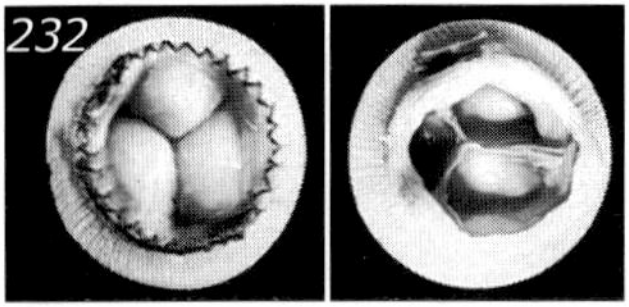

232

by Biomedica Mexicana; St Vincent *(Figure 233)* by Pacific Biomedical, Singapore; Wessex *(Figure 234)* by Wessex Medical Ltd, Sussex, UK; and Bravo *(Figure 235)* stented porcine xenograft by Bravo Cardiovascular, Inc, Irvine, California. The Shelhigh BioMitral valve (Shelhigh, Inc, Union, New Jersey) is a totally biological porcine valve as it has no fabric material. It has a composite construction using three carefully matched noncoronary porcine leaflets *(Figure 236)*. The stent is completely covered with pericardium, which is extended to form a sturdy sewing ring. It is subjected to the proprietary No-React detoxification and heparin treatment to facilitate cytocompatibility and inhibition of calcification.

The X–Cell porcine valve *(Figure 237)*, developed by St Jude Medical in conjunction with Hancock–Jaffe laboratories has innovative design features. These include a cell extraction process to selectively remove calcification sites from the porcine tissue, sterilisation by gamma irradiation, treatment to reduce leaflet stiffness and a cloth–free stent. It also undergoes zero-pressure fixation and, in smaller sizes, a composite leaflet arrangement. Clinical investigation with this prosthesis has begun.

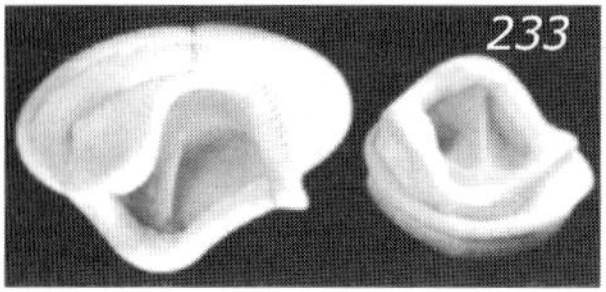

233

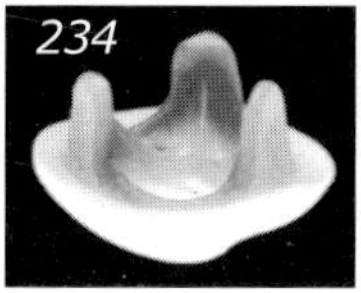

234

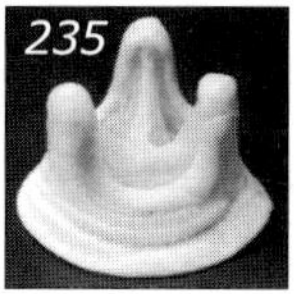

235

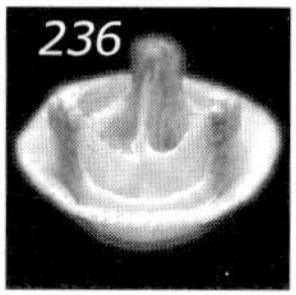

236

Valves harvested from kangaroos[128] and horses[129] have also been seriously considered for the fabrication of bioprosthetic valves. Dr Efstathios Andreas Agathos of the Medical-Psyhiko Clinic, Athens, Greece, during his tenure (as an associate of Dr Richard Engleman) at the Baystate Medical Center, Springfield, Massachusetts, proposed the use of marine mammal aortic or pulmonary valves (either stent-mounted or stentless) as xenografts (US Patent 6165216 0f 2000). Experimental studies in ovine and porcine models have been encouraging. Dr Jeffrey M Gross experimented with a carefully harvested porcine mitral valve (US Patent 5824067 of 1998).

237

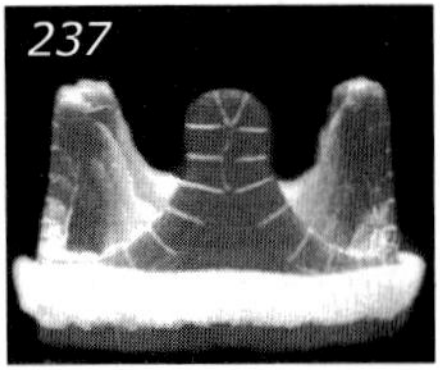

Stent-mounted homograft valves

Stent-mounted locally harvested aortic homografts failed to gain popularity because of the marked discrepancy in longevity between the free-hand sewn aortic homograft and the stented variety, ostensibly on account of the enhanced stress on the biological cusp tissue, leading to structural failure.[130] One of the reasons behind inevitable strucural failure has been attributed to the use of rigid stents[131] Nevertheless, a number of centres around the world have continued to patronise them, especially in the mitral position. In India, Dr AP Chaukar[132] and associates from the Lokmanya Tilak Memorial Hospital, Sion, Mumbai have been using such valves for several years *(Figure 238)*. They attribute [133] their

238

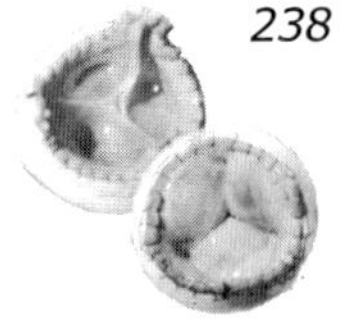

relative success to the use of specially fabricated highly flexible Delrin stents *(Figure 239)*.

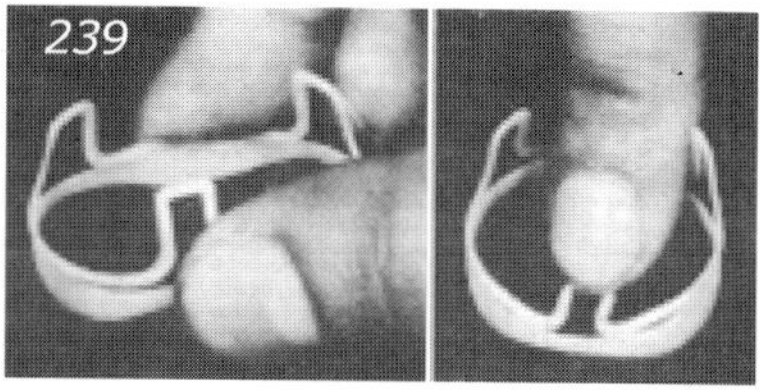

239

Stentless bioprosthetic valves

Stentless bioprosthetic valves include autografts, homografts, and stentless xenografts. They are devoid of any built-in support structure or bulky sewing ring. This gives them the advantage of a larger effective orifice area and superior haemodynamic efficiency, in comparison to standard stented or mechanical valves. They preserve the dynamic nature of the aortic annulus and retain the critical function of the sinuses of Valsalva in dissipating stress associated with valve closure. However the implantation of stentless valves is technically more challenging and less forgiving. They call for a learning curve packed with patience, discipline and the will to attain technical perfection.

Autografts are used for the Ross operation. The patient's own pulmonary valve is transferred to the aortic position, together with reconstruction the right ventricular outflow tract using a pulmonary homograft. Commercially processed porcine pulmonary valve such as the Cryolife–Ross xenograft *(Figure 240)* can also be used.

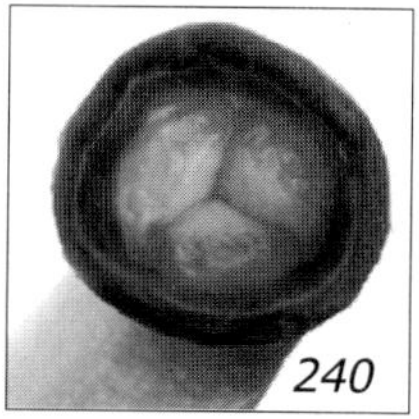

240

Several techniques are available for the preservation of cardiac allograft valves.[124] They include (i) lyophilised homografts which are nonviable and have

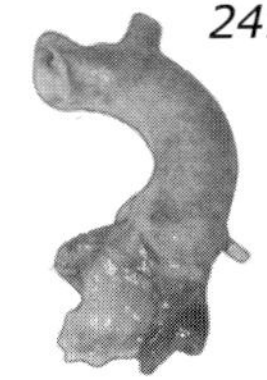

241

a disrupted histology; (ii) homovital homografts harvested under sterile condition and implanted within hours of retrieval; (iii) antibiotic-immersed fresh homografts which underwent progressive attenuation of viable cellular components; and (iii) cryopreserved, antibiotic-treated homograft valves harvested and processed under aseptic condition and frozen with dimethylsulphoxide. Cryopreserved (CryoLife Inc, Atlanta, Georgia) aortic *(Figure 241)*, mitral *(Figure 242)* and pulmonary *(Figure 243)* cadaver allografts, SJM–Lifenet allografts *(Figure 244)* and a few others are commercially available.

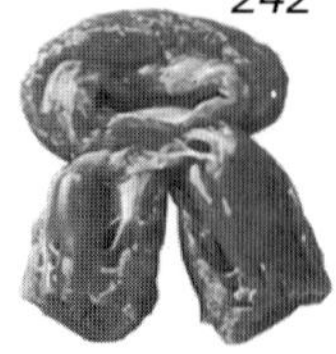

242

O'Brien's initial work between 1967 and 1972 was followed by a somewhat lengthy interlude till the concept of stentless xenografts was resurrected in 1988 by Dr Tirone E David and associates[134] of the Toronto General Hospital. They developed a prototype to improve haemodynamics, hoping for subsequent improvement in patient survival and valve durability. In support, the Framingham Heart Study averred that an increase in left ventricular hypertrophy was an important predictor of mortality.[135] Dr O Lund[136] of the Harefield Hospital, Middlesex, England demonstrated that the completeness of regression of left

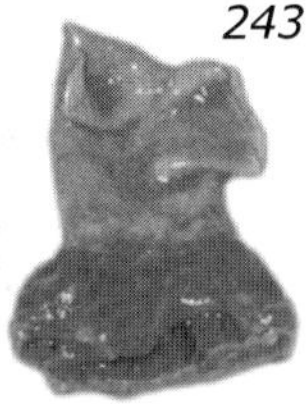

243

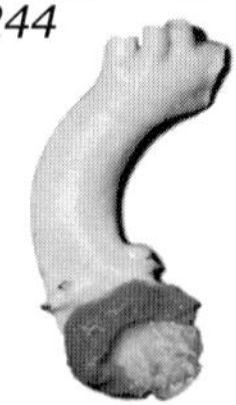

244

245

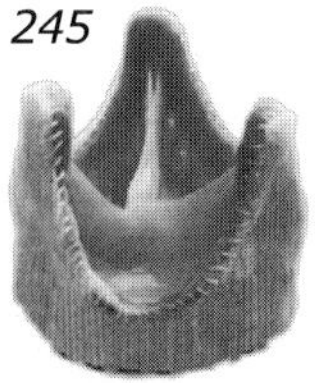

ventricular hypertrophy was the major factor determining late outcome following aortic valve replacement. These findings further consolidated interest in the stentless heterograft. David's initial experience led to the subsequent clinical availability and use of the St Jude Medical Toronto Stentless Porcine Valve *(Figure 245)*. Nicknamed the Toronto SPV valve, it is designed for subcoronary implantation. Its proximal sewing ring as well as the external surface, including the muscle shelf, are covered with fine Dacron mesh.

246

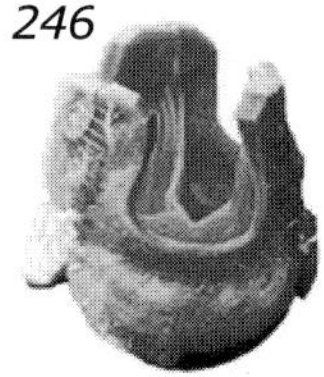

Leaving behind the era of formaldehyde fixation, O'Brien revived his composite stentless xenograft in 1991, this time using the modern technique of glutaraldehyde preservation. The Cryolife–O'Brien stentless bioprosthesis (also known as the O'Brien–Angell valve) is constructed using noncoronary leaflets obtained from three porcine valves *(Figure 246)*. The leaflets are carefully excised from valves already fixed in glutaraldehyde at zero-pressure. Individual noncoronary leaflets are then carefully matched for size and symmetry to assure competence and to aviod asynchronous opening. This promotes optimal leaflet coaption. The leaflets are sutured together along the free edges of the aortic wall at the commissures. The base of the valve is finished with a blanket stitch.The exclusion of any additional material, either biological or synthetic, at the annulus level of this xenograft aviods any unnecessary increase in its thickness or stiffness.

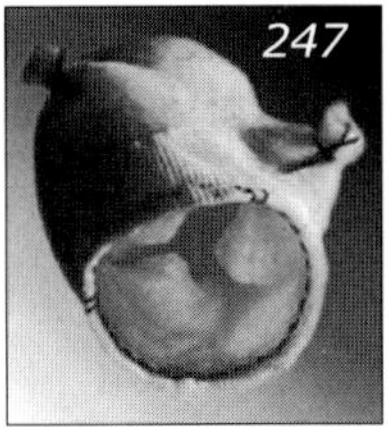

247

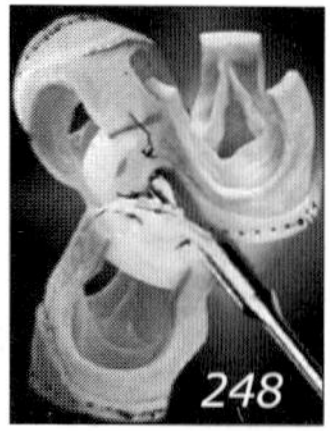

248

The Medtronic Freestyle valve *(Figure 247)* is a stentless porcine valve which incorporates a "total root" design. The valve can be implanted: (a) as a full root replacement where the entire native aortic root and valve are removed; (b) using a subcoronary technique; or (c) using a root inclusion technique where the prosthesis is implanted as a tube inside the native aorta. The valve is subjected to 'physiologic fixation'. The device undergoes antimineralisation treatment with alpha amino oleic acid. The 'Prestyled' Freestyle bioprosthesis *(Figure 248)* offers the convenience of a pre-trimmed version of the Freestyle aortic root bioprosthesis to match the surgeon's preferred implant technique. The use of an integrated holder system facilitates ease of handling during implantation.

The Baxter–Edwards Prima Stentless Porcine Bioprosthesis was also introduced in 1991, designed as a cylinder with prefashioned coronary openings. The prosthesis had a Dacron mesh that covered the muscle shelf, supported the coronary openings, and formed a thin proximal

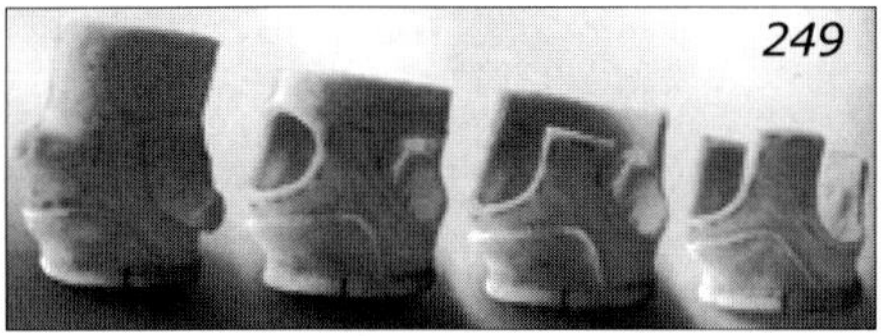

249

cuff. In 1996, a modified version called the Edwards Prima Plus Stentless Bioprosthesis *(Figure 249)* was introduced. This features a more versatile cylinder, unfashioned coronary

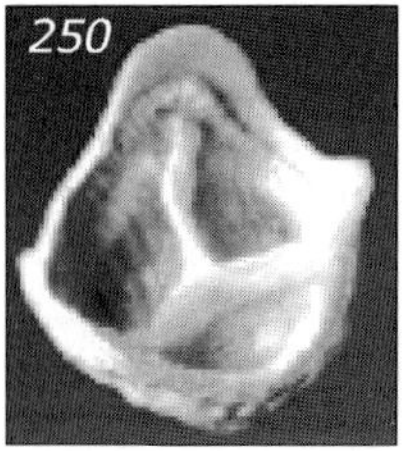

openings and Dacron mesh only over the muscle shelf and the proximal sewing cuff. The porcine tissue is glutaraldehyde-fixed at zero-pressure with sinus area dilatation. The prosthesis can be implanted by freehand subcoronary, miniroot cylinder or aortic root replacement technique.

The Biocor stentless porcine bioprosthesis *(Figure 250)* is a No–React treated Brazilian stentless valve with three individual porcine cusps to make a composite bioprosthesis, avoiding leaflets with muscular bands. The leaflets are fixed under zero-pressure and are sutured to a conduit of glutaraldehyde-treated bovine pericardium. The conduit is then shaped in a scalloped manner to mimic the natural aortic valve.

The Sorin Pericarbon Freedom pericardial bioprosthesis *(Figure 251)* is a stentless pericardial valve constructed from two separate sheets of glutaraldehyde-treated bovine pericardium. The first sheet is shaped to form the three leaflets by means of a process of atraumatic tissue fixation without the use of moulds. It is then sutured to the second sheet using a pyrolite carbon-coated suture. A 3 mm rim of pericardium beneath the pericardial cusps accommodates the inflow suture line. The suture line is especially designed to dampen the mechanical stress at the level of the commissures. The outflow of the valve is partially scalloped, although further trimming is usually necessary beneath the coronary arteries.

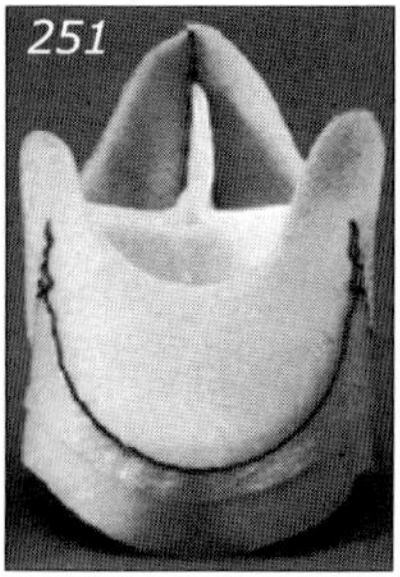

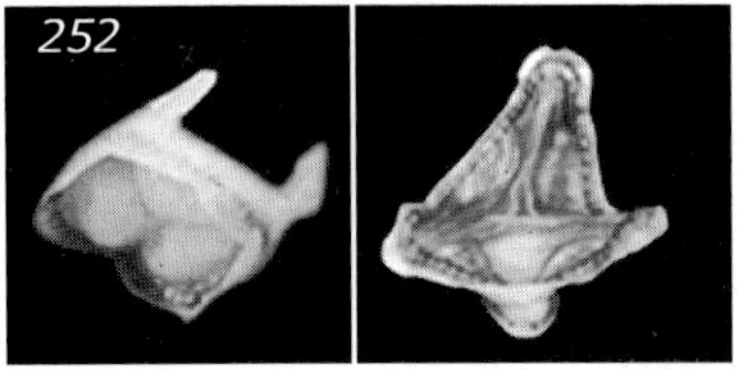

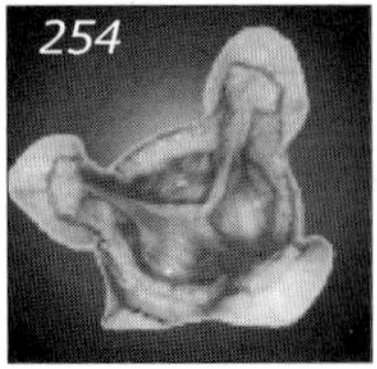

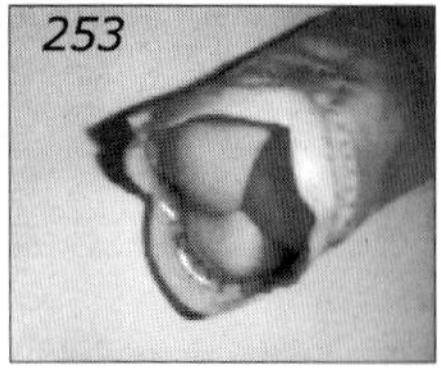

The Shelhigh standard stentless aortic valve is constructed from three separate porcine non-coronary cusps, put together in a unique fashion and then covered with pericardium. It is treated with the proprietary No-React anticalcification treatment. The device is claimed to be distortion-resistant with assured coaptation even when distended up to 3 mm in diameter *(Figure 252)*. The Shelhigh SuperStentless "skeletonised" valve *(Figure 253)* is claimed to be always competent like stented bioprostheses. It allows oversizing even in asymmetric aortic root as no sutures are needed in the vicinity of the cornary ostia. The extended tissue averts accidental cuspal damage. The product is stored in benzyl alcohol, obviating the need for vigorous rinsing. It also comes with an extended pericardial cuff *(Figure 254)* to allow a mini-root implantation.

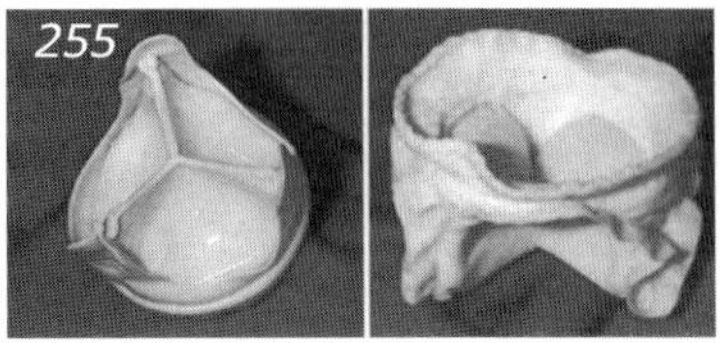

The Braile bovine pericardium stentless valve *(Figure 255)* is manufactured with bovine pericardium and Braile porcine stentless valve *(Figure 256)* from suitable porcine aortic valves. Both are treated with glutaraldehyde at zero–

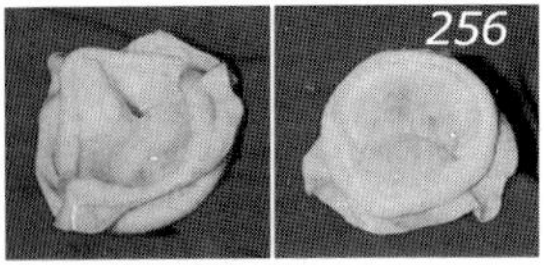
256

pressure. Braille–Bentall conduits *(Figure 257)* for aortic root replacement and pericardial valved conduit *(Figure 258)*

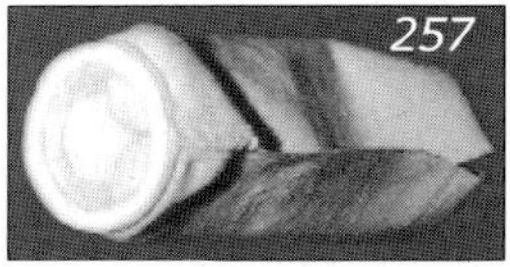
257

also received surgeons' attention. Braile porcine valve cuspids *(Figure 259)* made from porcine aortic valve and cuspid of bovine pericardium *(Figure 260)*, treated with glutaraldehyde and preserved in formaldehyde are also available. Baruah, too, had designed a stentless bovine pericardial aortic valve *(Figure 261).* Baruah anatomically composed aortic and pulmonary valves *(Figure 262)* were also available for some time.

The Quattro valve is a quadricusp stentless mitral bioprosthesis conceptualised by Frater[137] in 1991. The name refers to its four-leaflet configuration. Fabricated completely of bovine pericardial tissue, the valve incorporates a full subvalvular apparatus that maintains the mitral annular-papillary continuity *(Figure 263)*. It is designed to have one large anterior and one posterior leaflet consisting of 3 scallops. All pieces are aligned by non-load-bearing sutures. The sewing ring consists of 2

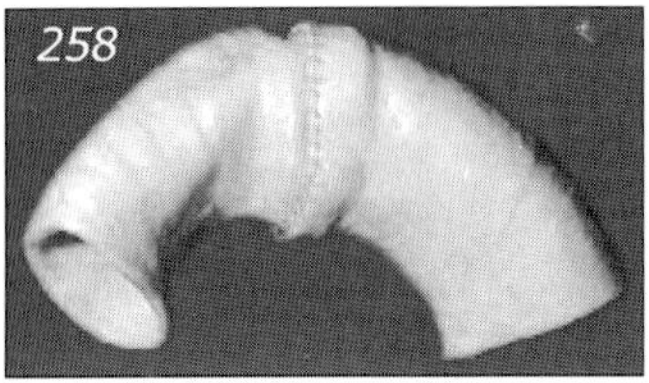
258

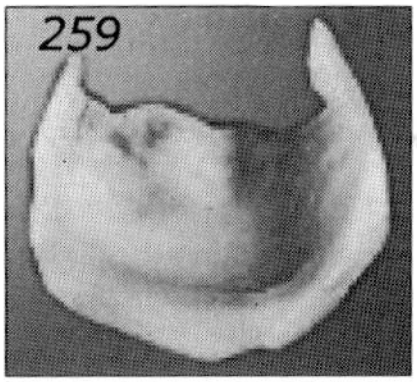
259

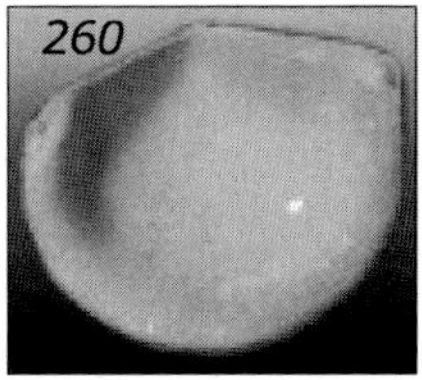
260

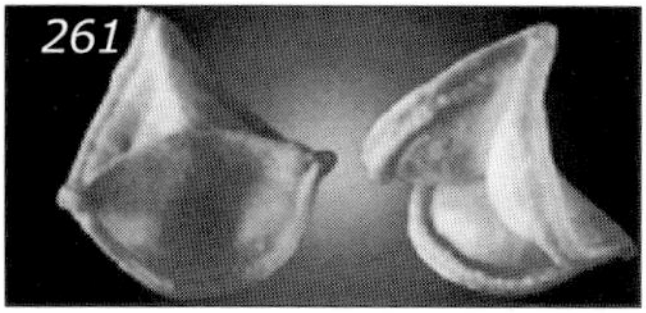

layers of pericardium and thus can function as an annuloplasty ring There are 2 joint papillary flaps at the anterolateral and postero-medial sides. Each papillary flap supports the anterior as well as the posterior leaflet. The annulus is D–shaped, and during valve closure, the anterior leaflet meets the other 3 scallops.[138]

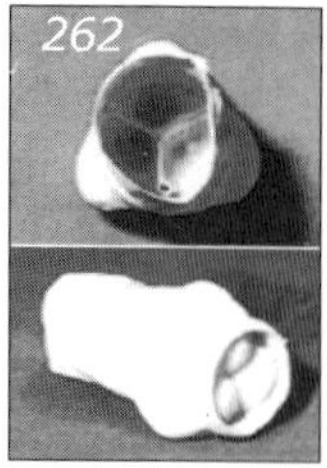

The pericardium is tanned by glutaraldehyde for collagen cross-linking and for removal of immunogenecity. Residual aldehydes known to be responsible for tissue calcification are capped by additional treatment with a liquid polyol based anticalcification treatment (US patent 5476516 of 1995). This anticalcification treatment, EnCap, has proven efficient over a 4 to 6 year period in a younger subset of patients (personal communication: Dr Frater). It is designed to be relatively easy to implant as compared with other stentless valves. Human clinical trials have been carried out in Europe, South Africa, the Middle East, and Canada, with encouraging performance and patient outcomes. Recently, marketing rights of this product have been taken over by Glycar Inc, Bronxville, New York and SJM Quattro is now known as Glycar Quattro.

Baruah stentless mitral valve prostheses *(Figure 264)* were anatomically designed prostheses with chordae meant to be brought out of the veft ventricular apex for fixation. The initial few valves were implanted at the Prince of Wales

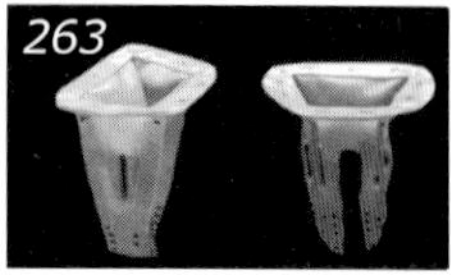

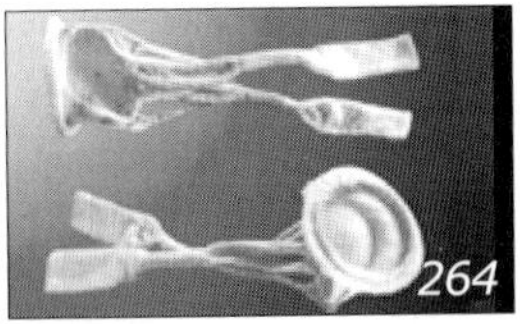

264

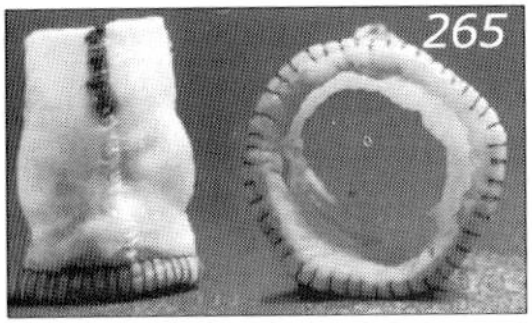

265

Hospital, Chinese University, Hong Kong by Dr Jonathan Ho in 1992. Subsequently these valves were implanted in a few Indian institutions. Their production was discontinued after a few years for undeclared reasons.

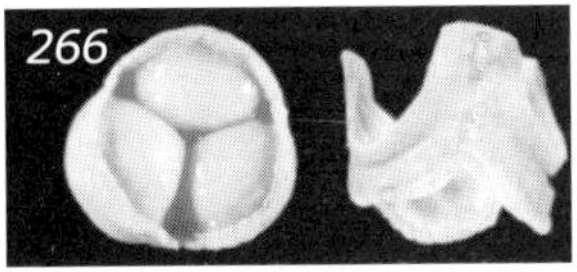

266

The CarboMedics Oxford Photofix stentless *(Figure 265)* valve is a composite xenograft root constructed from three selected porcine noncoronary cusps fixed by the photofix process. The valve inflow has a low pericardial cuff. Consequently there are no coronaries, cloth, or muscle bar in the structure. It is made from a biostable collagenous soft pliable tissue with greater resistance to calcification than glutaraldehyde-treated tissue.[139]

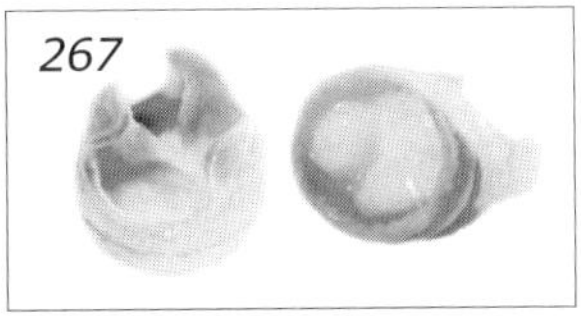

267

Several other innovative stentless porcine aortic valves,[140] viz, the Unique Suture Line stentless valve (Biosud S.A., Buenos Aires, Argentina), Labcor (Labcor Laboratories, Belo Horizonte, Brazil), currently marketed by Sulzer Medica as Synergy Stentless *(Figure 266),* Aortech Elan stentless valve *(Figure 267),* Conforma (Heartline, UK) stentless valve and Xenolife stentless are among other stentless bioprostheses showcased.

The Medtronic Contegra pulmonary valved conduit bioprosthesis consists of a heterologous bovine jugular vein with a tri-leaflet venous valve and a natural sinus slightly larger in diameter than its lumen. The conduit is preserved in buffered glutaraldehyde solution in a concentration low enough to preserve the flexibility of the leaflet material. It is indicated for implantation in children and young adults for the correction of right ventricular outflow tract obstruction; pulmonary valve replacement during Ross procedure; replacement of previously implanted but dysfunctional pulmonary homograft or a failed pulmonary prosthesis.

The Horizon ...and Beyond

The currently available prosthetic valves come as a mixed package of boon and bane. Mechanical valves require the use of anticoagulants, which are expensive, need changes in the patient's lifestyle, and are replete with fears of haemolytic, thrombotic, embolic or haemorrhagic complications; or worse, a catastrophic device dysfunction. Bioprosthetic valves do not require systemic anticoagulation but are prone to calcification and degeneration, and hence often not an option for younger patients. Further, neither type of valve has the potential for growth or repair. Thus many children and young adults, who have undergone valve replacement surgery, are forced to undergo repeat procedures during their lifetimes. Under such circumstances, the incessant quest for an 'ideal' heart valve substitute would appear to be utopian. But the ingenuity of the human mind, persistently and perseveringly pursuing the permutations and combinations of plausible alternatives, has risen to the occasion with exciting alternatives, among which the domain of tissue engineering has evinced enormous promise.

Tissue-engineered heart valves

Tissue engineering of heart valves is a relatively recent but rapidly expanding subject engaging biomedical scientists. Its objective is to fabricate a viable and functional heart valve from autologous cells. The

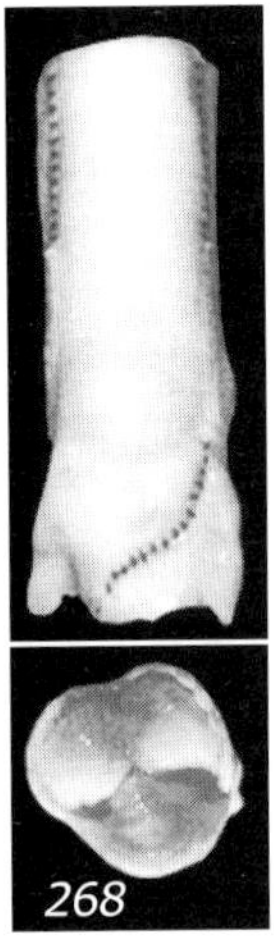

268

basic idea is to transplant autologous cells onto a biocompatible and biodegradable scaffold that is shaped like a heart valve. Once the cells have become attached to the scaffold, they form their own extracellular matrix while the polymer scaffold starts to degrade. With this approach, it is theoretically possible to generate a viable and autologous tissue-engineered heart valve that can be implanted into the same patient from whom the cells were harvested. Such an implantable tissue-engineered structure would have certain potential advantages over the conventional heart valve substitutes. A valve that would eliminate the need for lifelong anticoagulants, would not calcify, and would provide for long-term durability as well as growth, is the ultimate goal for researchers in the area of tissue engineering.

Native valves are primarily populated with two different types of cells. The first cell type is the valvular interstitial cell, which is responsible for matrix synthesis and repair within the leaflets. Several institutions are currently working to characterise these unique cells. The second type of cell present is the endothelial cell, which forms a monolayer on the leaflet surface and provides a haemocompatible blood-contacting surface. While both cell types are necessary to create a tissue-engineered valve, other approaches are being investigated to achieve this objective.

The first such approach involves a biological or synthetic scaffold that would be populated with the patient's cells *in vivo*. The CryoLife SynerGraft valve *(Figure 268)* is the best example of this approach. It is a decellularised and cryopreserved xenogenic stentless valve which utilises non-cross-linked tissue.[141] Initially, as a novel tissue engineering approach to improving replacement heart valve durability, a decellularisation process was developed to replace the use of cross-linking to limit xenograft antigenicity. Stentless bioprosthetic valves were fabricated from acellular tissues, cryopreserved, sterilised, and then implanted as pulmonary valve replacements, in sheep to start with. In human subjects, reconstruction of the right ventricular outflow tract was performed by Dr MJF Bechtel and colleagues at the University Hospital, Luebeck, Germany. The initial clinical experience has been gratifying.[142]

Cross-linked xenogenic tissues are also being investigated for their ability to promote host cell repopulation *in vivo*. Sulzer Medica's proprietary photo-oxidized bovine pericardium (CardioFix), a decellularised material experimentally shown to be noncytotoxic and nonimmunogenic, is one such tissue. St Jude Medical is investigating detoxification treatments for glutaraldehyde cross-linked tissue and subsequent modifications to promote cell adhesion and migration. Decellularised xenogenic valves have the obvious advantage of possessing the proper matrix architecture. Several groups are working on seeding these valves with autologous fibroblastic and endothelial cells.

An alternate approach to creating a tissue-engineered valve involves the *in vitro* cell seeding of either synthetic or biological scaffolds. In one preliminary study where such seeded constructs were implanted in the pulmonary position in sheep, good valve function was observed at the end of one month.

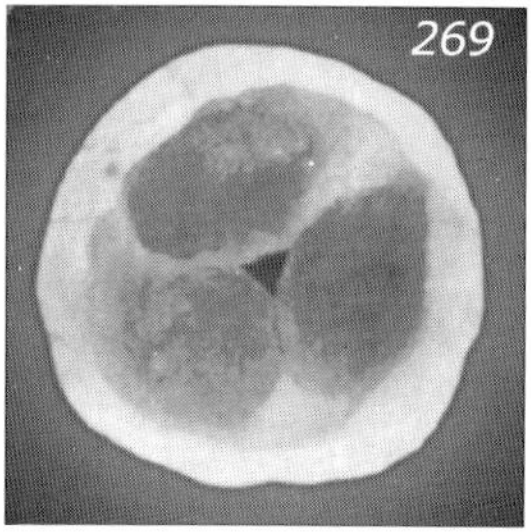

Others are investigating the use of degradable polymer scaffolds. *In vitro* experiments in this direction were initially commenced with single leaflets before progressing to complete valves in a project undertaken at the Boston Children Hospital. Trileaflet heart valves were fabricated from novel bioabsorbable polymers and sequentially seeded with autologous ovine myofibroblasts and endothelial cells.[143] Animal experiments have been unequivocally encouraging, with echocardiographically demonstrable mobile functioning leaflets without stenosis, thrombus or aneurysm up to 20 weeks. A uniform, layered cuspal tissue with endothelium was seen on histological examination and a confluent smooth valvular surface on electron microscopy. Mechanical properties were comparable with those of native tissues at 20 weeks *(Figure 269)*. Complete degradation of the polymers occurred by 8 weeks.

The type of scaffold material is of crucial importance, because it has to meet many requirements. It has to be strong enough to withstand high blood pressure, has to provide anchorage points for cells to hold on to and has to support the developing tissue to form extracellular matrix. It also has to take care of the transport of nutrients and waste products and has to stimulate blood vessel ingrowth and angiogenesis. The scaffold also has to be porous, elastic, biodegradable, biocompatible and easy to process.

Polymers

A prosthetic valve constructed with polymeric leaflets has durability superior to that of biological valves. It is haemocompatible, does not require systemic anticoagulation and should prove to be a boon in the quest for a perfect valve. Although the design of such a polymer valve would appear to be a relatively straightforward exercise, earlier efforts in this direction have been disappointing. However, the use of polymers as raw material for valve construction is currently experiencing a phase of renaissance. Because synthetic polymers such as polyurethanes possess high tensile strength and excellent resistance to cyclic fatigue, this class of materials has been widely studied as a potential prosthetic heart valve material. Researchers from the Pennsylvania State University described a prosthetic polymer heart valve fabricated with leaflets of polyetherurethane urea (Biomer, Ethicon, Somerville, New Jersey). While their valve, evaluated in the ovine mitral model,[144] provided a model system for testing materials, its success was ultimately limited by its design. Valves fabricated with leaflets of Biomer and other proprietary materials, were evaluated for thrombosis, calcification and durability. It was found that valve designs that minimise leaflet stress and areas of stasis may be more conducive to preventing thrombus formation and increasing durability. The possible advantage of surface modification to prevent thrombosis has also been recognised. Innovative design combined with anti-thrombogenic surface treatments may soon lead to a non-thrombogenic, durable polymer valve.

Many researchers are devotedly engaged in exploring the superlative scope of polymers and allied materials for heart valve prostheses.

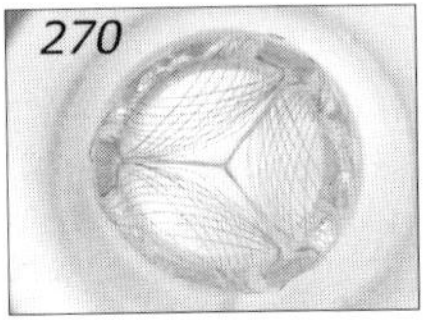

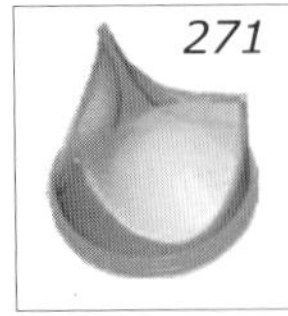

Dr Richard T Schoephoerster of the Cardiovascular Research Center, Florida International University, in collaboration with Dr Vladimir Kasyanov from Latvia, and other research workers, is working on a novel artificial heart valve design that incorporates a composite material, polypropylene threads embedded in polyurethane, with the thread configuration mimicking *in vivo* collagen architecture *(Figure 270)*. Researchers at AorTech are in the advanced stage of developing a new generation, synthetic, trileaflet heart valve provisionally christened Tri–Leaflet *(Figure 271)*. During the research and development stages, the device had initially been fabricated from Elast–Eon, a siloxane-impregnated polymer developed by Dr Pathiraja A Gunatillake, a molecular scientist of Sri Lankan origin. Currently the material used is Peek–Optima, a semicrystalline polymer (polyaryletherketone) manufactured by Invibio, Lancashire, UK. This material is claimed to be immensely durable and versatile. Peek–Optima is claimed to have undergone rigorous biocompatibility and biostability assay to ensure its suitability for implantation. The Leeds University group, headed by Professor John Fisher of the Department of Mechnical Engineering, also has extensive experience in the field, and has been involved with the development of polyurethane heart valves *(Figure 272)*. Another valve called Coraflex *(Figure 273)* is being tried out by Biocontrol Technology Inc.

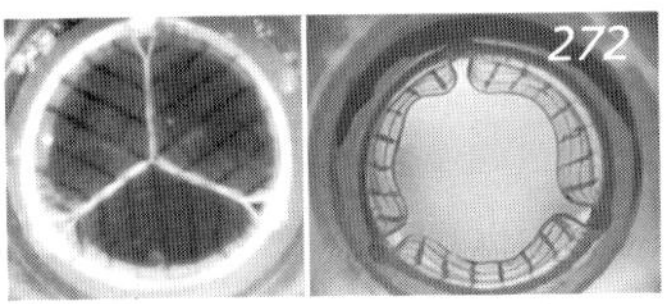

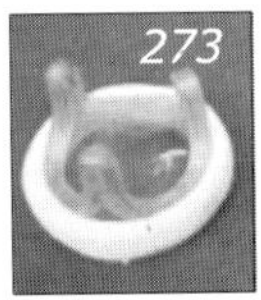

Flexible tubes as heart valves

Dr James L Cox, during his tenure at the Barnes Hospital, St Louis, Missouri, first drew attention to the conceptual link between the formation of heart valves in man and how mature heart valves function. He propounded that since the cardiovascular system begins in utero as a simple tube, the connections between atria and ventricles, as well as those between the ventricles and great vessels, remain in tubular form all through. As the heart enlarges, the non-essential portions of these embryological tubes dissolve, leaving behind only the functional remnants of the tubular walls. Between the atria and ventricles, these tubular remnants become the leaflets and chordae tendineae of the mitral and tricuspid valves. Between the ventricles and great vessels, they take the shape of the aortic and pulmonic valvar cusps. Hence, on attaining maturity, all four of the heart's native valves function as simple tubes whose sides collapse when exposed to external pressure.

Thus came into existence the concept of heart valve replacement using flexible tubes (US patent 5480424 of 1996). The 3F aortic bioprosthesis is a tubular-design, biological heart valve fabricated from three equal leaflets of equine pericardium processed with proprietary formulations of buffered glutaraldehyde. Each leaflet has been cut by means of a proprietary computer-aided process that ensures precise reproducibility from leaflet to leaflet. The valve is then assembled in a tubular shape, with unique locking stitches that result in a secure attachment of the commissural tabs *(Figure 274).*

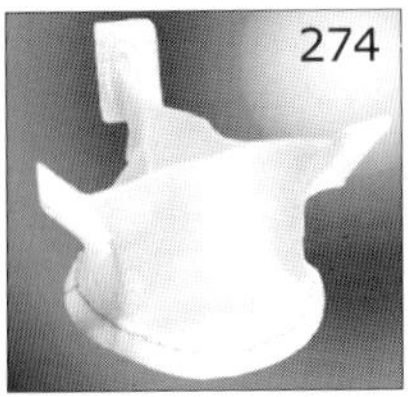

274

Bypassing the surgeon

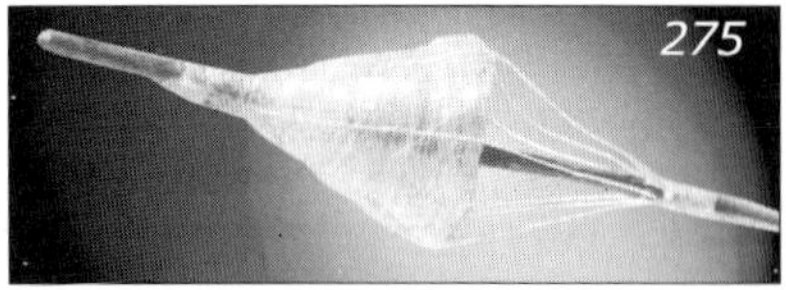
275

In all probability, the practical concept of a catheter-mounted aortic valve originated way back in 1965 when Dr H Davies[145] described a cone-shaped valve *(Figure 275)*, used experimentally in dogs. Dr SD Moulopoulos and associates from the Department of Clinical Therapeutics at the Alexandra Hospital, Athens, Greece submitted three designs of catheter-mounted aortic valves.[146] Two of these were in the form of balloons and one in the shape of an umbrella. In their canine experiments these polyurethane valves were positioned just distal to the coronary ostia. Dr Richard L Dobben conceptualised (US Patent 4994077 of 1991) a disc-shaped flap valve threaded on a bent wire meant to be anchored to the aorta with the help of a clip or a stent *(Figure 276)*. In 1992, Dr RR Andersen and colleagues[147] from the Skejby University Hospital, Aarhus, Denmark undertook animal experiments to implant a catheter-mounted expandable stent encasing an intact porcine aortic valve. Dr George P Teitelbaum proposed a thermosensitive, percutaneously inserted cardiac valve *(Figure 277)*. "A cardiac valve implanted within the heart is given where an expansible valve

276

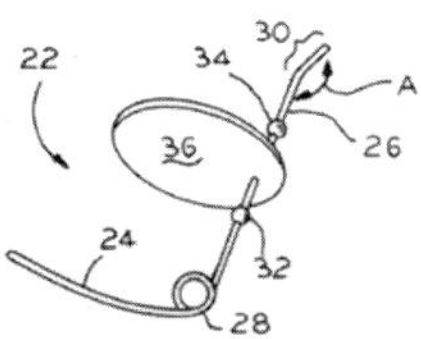

277

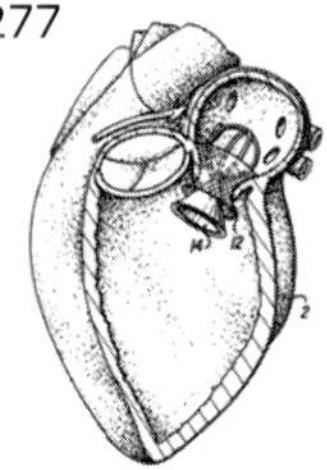

maintained in a collapsed form by cold temperature is percutaneously inserted along a releasable guide- wire in a cooled sheath and when positioned is expanded by withdrawing the cold temperature [sic]," read the abstract in US Patent 5332402 of 1994.

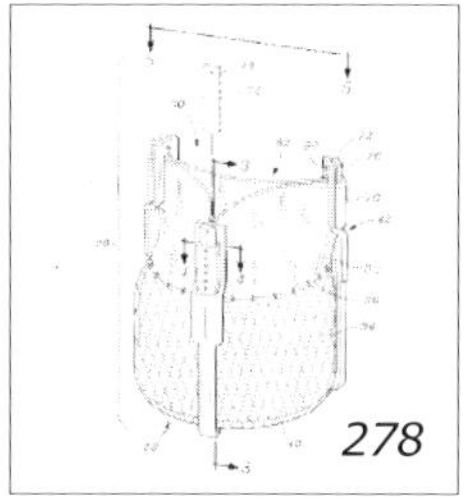

278

The idea was revived in the closing years of the twentieth century. Dr Stefan Schrek, under the auspices of Edwards Lifesciences, conceptualised an expandable, preassembled annular base with multiple upstanding commissure posts *(Figure 278)*, the multileaflet fabric subassembly being attached to the base (US Patent 6454799 of 2000). Drs Y Boudjemline and P Bonhoeffer[148] from the Service de Cardiologie Pediatrique, Hôpital Necker Enfants Malades, Paris had reported their experience with transcatheter implantation of a bovine valve in pulmonary position in lambs in 2002. Later they applied this technique in a 12–year–old boy with valvular dysfunction in a right ventricle to pulmonary artery prosthetic conduit.[149] Subsequently they used a bovine jugular vein containing a valve sutured into a stent *(Figure 279)* and performed aortic valve replacement through a percutaneous technique in lambs.[150]

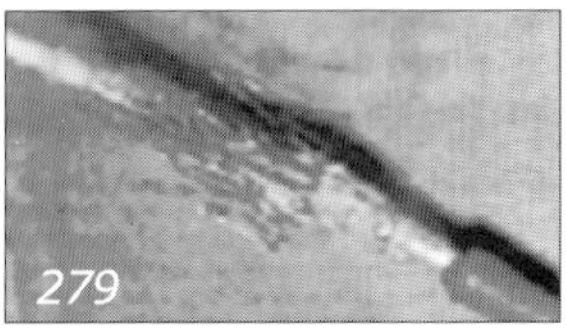

279

Dr Sinan Muftu and other research workers at the Northeastern College of Engineering, Boston, Massachussetts, innovated a prototype of a collapsible copper wire frame and latex glove fingers *(Figure 280)* to demonstrate the working of such a system with artificial

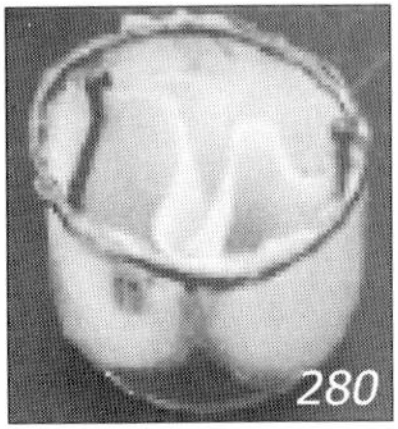

280

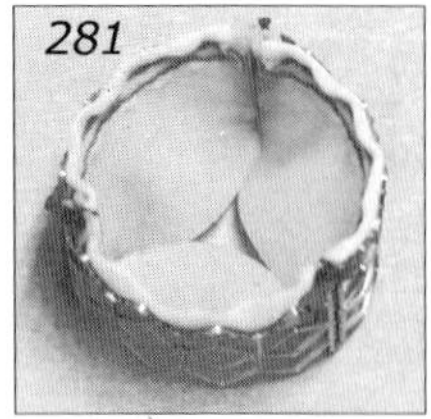

281

material. Other groups have also been enthusiastically working in this direction. Dr Alain Cribier and colleagues from the Charles Nicolle Hospital, Rouen, France developed a percutaneous implantable prosthetic heart valve composed of 3 bovine pericardial leaflets mounted within a balloon-expandable stent *(Figure 281)*. After in vitro testing and animal experiments, in April 2002, the first human implantation was successfully performed in a 57–year–old man with calcific aortic stenosis, cardiogenic shock, subacute leg ischaemia, and other associated noncardiac diseases.[151] Recently Dr Troy R Norred of Columbia, Missouri obtained a patent for a percutaneously implantable aortic valve with an extended expandable stent system *(Figure 282)* for the ascending aorta (US Patent 6482228 of 2002) for secure retention of the device.

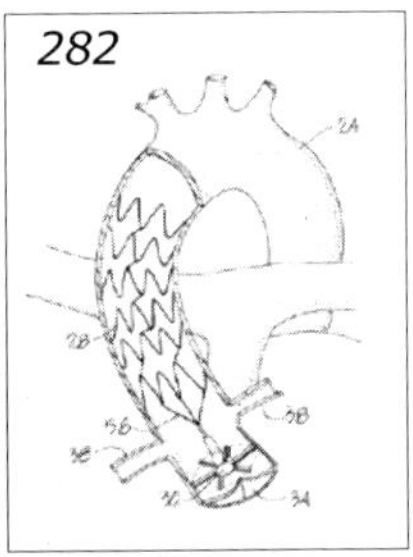

282

Recently, Dr Robert V Snyders obtained a patent (US Patent 6540782 of 2003) for a catheter-mounted, multicuspid prosthesis with a flexibly resilient frame *(Figure 283)*, sized and shaped for insertion in a position between the upstream region and the downstream region of the damaged valve. The device has multiple anchors for fixation. Attached to the frame is a flexible valve element which moves to an open or closed position in accordance with intracardiac haemodynamics.

On the anvil

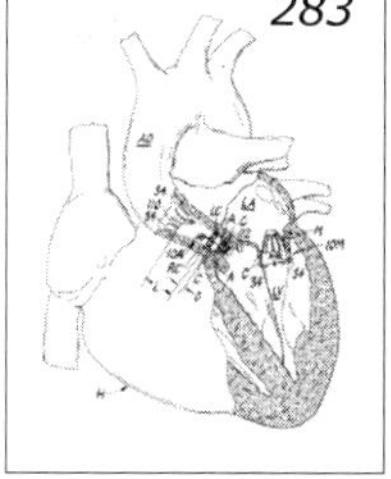

283

The wizard of fibreoptics, Dr James D Byrne, conceptualised an optic fibre heart valve prosthesis *(Figure 284)*. Trileaflet metallic valve designs were initially patented by Bokros and Jonathan C Stupka (US Patent 5843183 of 1998). Drs Didier Lapeyre of France and Ulrich Steinseifer of Denmark fabricated an improved version (US Patent 6395024 of 2002). Dr Michael Philip Goldowsky blueprinted a valve based on the torsion principle (US Patent 6432135 of 2002). Dr Roberto Pedros innovated a novel stapling device for valve implantation (US Patent 6413274 of 2002). Dr Dongbu Cao patented a flexible heart valve with movable commissures (US Patent 6461382 of 2002). Mario Osvaldo Vrandecic Peredo (US Patent 6409759 of 2002) proposed extended sewing rims for harvested tissue valves. This principle was extended to cryopreserved and other stentless tissue valves by Dr David H Adams (US Patent 6540781 of 2003). Very recently Carpentier and others patented a highly flexible stent which would lend unprecedented flexibility to valves fabricated on them (US Patent 6558418 of 2003).

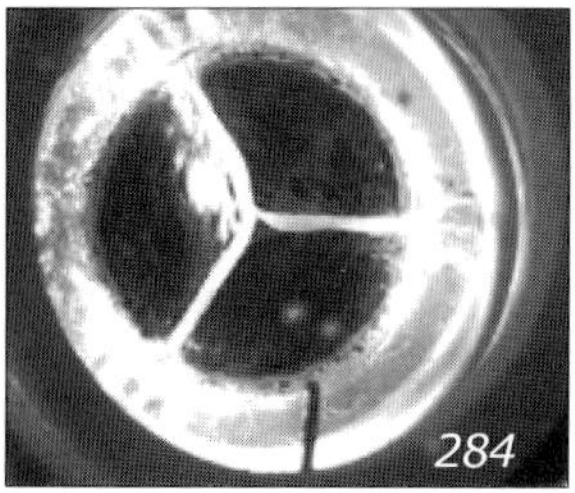

284

A quadrileaflet mechanical prosthetic aortic valve[152] is also on the anvil. The leaflets have rods extendihg at either end of their base. Each end lies in a niche carved in the valve housing, allowing the leaflets to open up to an

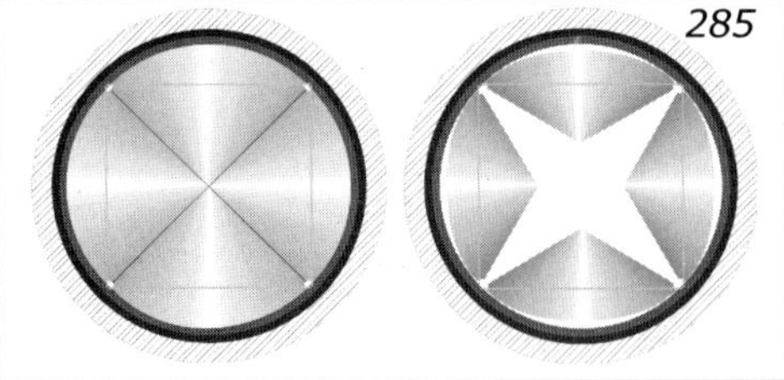
285

angle of about 75 degrees, thereby facilitating central blood flow during systole and easy closure during diastole. Tiny gaps at these points when the valve is closed are meant to keep the pivotal area constantly irrigated with blood without producing any significant regurgitation *(Figure 285).* The device is awaiting fabrication and a patent.

For the moment it seems that designing the ideal prosthetic heart valve is likely to occupy the visionary for many years to come. If human ingenuity is ever able to achieve absolute perfection in this matter, a new set of issues will emerge to be debated by the medical profession. Foremost among those will be the ethical questions regarding accessibility and availability of artificial valve devices for underprivileged patients around the globe. The heft of the price tag and the associated need for investments in research and development will underscore the predicament of those who must make medical decisions. Under such circumstances, it is the governments of developing nations that should take up the cudgel for the have–nots. They must devise fail–safe mechanisms to subsidise the medical expenses of those living on the edge of society. If that can be accomplished, it would be the best possible tribute to all those who have crusaded against valvular heart disease.

References

1. Hufnagel CA, Harvey WP. The surgical correction of aortic insufficiency. Bull Georgetown Univ Med Cent 1953; 6: 60–63.

2. Schwartz DC, Kaplan S. The caged ball valve circa 1858. Am J Cardiol 1966; 18: 942.

3. Campbell JM. an artificial aortic valve : preliminary report. J Thorac Surg 1950; 19: 312–318.

4. Lam CR, Aram HH, Munnel ER. An experimental study of aortic valve homografts. Surg Gynecol Obstet 1952; 94: 129–135.

5. Murray G. Homologous aortic-valve-segment transplants as surgical treatment for aortic and mitral insufficiency. Angiology 1956; 7: 466–471.

6. Lower RR, Stofer RC, Shumway NE. A study of pulmonary valve autotransplantation. Surgery 1960; 48: 1090–1100.

7. Lower RR, Stofer RC, Shumway NE. Total excision of the mitral valve and replacement with the autologous pulmonic valve. J Thorac Cardiovasc Surg 1961; 42: 696–706.

8. Denton GR. A plastic prosthesis [without moving parts] for the atrio-ventricular valves. Proceedings of the Surgical Forum

Sessions of the XXXVI Clinical Congress, Am Coll Surgeons, 1950. Philadelphia: W B.Saunders, 1951: 239–245.

9. Harken DE, Black H, Ellis LB, Dextel I. The surgical correction of mitral insufficiency. J Thorac Surg 1954; 28: 604–627.

10. Harken DE. Heart valves: ten commandments and still counting. Ann Thorac Surg 1989; 48 [Suppl]: S18–S19.

11. Norman AF. The first mitral valve replacement. Ann Thorac Surg 1991; 51: 525–526.

12. Lewis FJ, Tauftc M. Closure of atrial septal defects with the aid of hypothermia: experimental accomplishments and the report of one successful case. Surgery 1953; 33: 52–59.

13. Lillehei CW, Gott VL, De Wall RA, Varco RL. Surgical correction of pure mitral insufficiency by anuloplasty under direct vision. Lancet 1957; 77: 446–449.

14. Hufnagel CA, Vilkgas PD, Nahas H. Experiences with new types of aortic valvular prostheses. Ann Surg 1958; 147: 636–645.

15. Edwards WS, Smith L. Aortic valve replacement with a subcoronary ball valve. Surg Forum 1958; 9: 309–313.

16. Roe BB. A compression-molded leaflet prosthetic valve. Ann Thorac Surg, 1989; 48 [Suppl]: S26–S27.

17. Kay EB, Suzuki A. Evolution of aortic valvular prostheses. J Thorac Cardiovasc Surg 1963; 45: 372–381.

18. Bahnson HT, Spencer FC, Busse EFG, Davis FW Jr. Cusp replacement and coronary artery perfusion in open operations on the aortic valve. Ann Surg 1960; 152: 494–505.

19. Roe BB, Owsley JW, Boudoures PC. Experimental results with a prosthetic aortic valve. J Thorac Cardiovasc Surg 1958; 36: 563–570.

20. Roe BB, Burke MF, Zebner H Jr. The subcoronary implantation of a flexible tricuspid aortic valve prosthesis. J Thorac Cardiovasc Surg, 1960; 40: 561–567.

21. van der Spuy JC. Considerations in the prosthetic construction of the aortic valve. S Afr Med J 1964; 38: 768–770.

22. Harken DE, Soroff HS, Taylor WJ. Lefemine AA, Gupta SK, Lanzer S. Partial and complete prostheses in aortic insufficiency. J Thorac Cardiovasc Surg 1960; 40: 744–762.

23. Harken DE. I. A new caged-ball aortic and mitral valve and II. Monitoring and controlled respiration In critically ill patients. J Mt Sinai Hosp 1965; 32: 93–106.

24. McGoon DC, Moffitt EA. Total prosthetic reconstruction of the aortic valve. J Thorac Cardiovasc Surg 1963; 46: 162–173.

25. Kernan MC, Newman MM, Levowitz BS, Stuckey JH, Dennis C. J Thorac Surg 1957; 33: 698–706.

26. Ellis FH Jr., Bulbulian AH. Prosthetic replacement of the mitral valve: Preliminary experimental observations. Mayo Clinic Proceedings 1958; 33: 532–534.

27. Paton BC. Discussion in: McGregor RR, Braley SA. Methods of preparing silastic for prostheses. In Merendino KA, Ed. Prosthetic Valves for Cardiac Surgery. Springfield: Charles C Thomas, 1961; 172–198.

28. Schwab L. Discussion in: Stuckey JH,Newman MM, Berg E, Goodman S, Dennis C. Design and placement of prosthetic valves to fit in the mitral ring of the dog after excision of the leaflets. In Merendino KA, Ed: Prosthetic Valves for Cardiac Surgery. Springfield: Charles C Thomas, 1961; 266–285.

29. Berg EH, Goodman SE, Stuckey JH, Newman ME. Total replacement of the mitral valve. Surg Forum 1957; 8: 363–367.

30. Frater RWM, Ellis FH Jr. Problems in the development of a mitral valve prosthesis. In Merendino KA, Ed: Prosthetic Valves for Cardiac Surgery. Springfield: Charles C Thomas, 1961; 244–265.

31. Doumanian AV, Ellis FH. Prolonged survival after total replacement of the mitral valve in dogs. J Thorac Cardiovasc Surg 1961; 42: 683–695.

32. Akutsu T, Dreyer B, Kolff WJ. Polyurethane artificial heart valves in animals. J Appl Physiol 1959; 14: 1045–1048.

33. Akutsu T, Mirkovitch V, Kolff WJ. Teflon as experimental replacement for mitral and tricuspid valves. J Surg Research 1961; 1: 188–191.

34. Barnard CN, McKenzie MB, Schrire V. A surgical approach to mitral insufficiency. Br J Surg 1961; 48: 655–662.

35. van der Spuy JC. Considerations in the prosthetic construction of a completely anatomical whole mitral valve from autogenous tissues. S Afr Med J 1964; 38: 771–775.

36. Ross DN. The replacement of the aortic valve with biological tissue. Ann Thorac Surg 1968; 5: 383–392.

37. Frater RWM, Berghuis J, Brown AL Jr, Ellis FH Jr. The experimental and clinical use of autogenous pericardium for the replacement and extension of mitral and tricuspid valve cusps and chordae. J Cardiovasc Surg [Torino] 1965; 6: 214–228.

38. Frater RWM, Berghüis J, Brown AL Jr, Ellis FH Jr. Autogenous pericardium for posterior mitral leaflet replacement. Surgery 1963; 54: 260–268.

39. Barnard CN, Schrire V. Ivalon baffle for posterior leaflet replacement in the treatment of mitral valve insufficiency: a follow-up study. Surgery 1968; 63: 727–730.

40. Braunwald NS, Cooper T, Morrow AG. Complete replacement of the mitral valve: successful clinical application of a flexible polyurethane prosthesis. J Thorac Cardiovasc Surg 1960; 40: 1–11.

41. Westaby S. Landmarks in Cardiac Surgery. Oxford: Isis Medical Media, 1997.

42. Derloshon G. One for the Heart. Irvine: Shiley Incorporated, 1983: 94.

43. Matthews AM. The development of the Starr–Edwards heart valve. Tex Heart Inst J 1998; 25: 282–293.

44. Gott Vl, Daggett Rl, Whiffen Jd, Koepke De, Rowe Gg, Young WP. A hinged-leaflet valve for total replacement of the human aortic valve. J Thorac Cardiovasc Surg 1964; 48: 713–725.

45. Cooley DA, Liotta D, Cromie HW, Hall CW, Wieting DW, Bloodwell RD. Aortic valve prosthesis incorporating ligthweight titanium ball, Dacron velour covered cage and seat. Trans Amer Soc Artif Int Organs 1967;13:93.

46. Campbell A, Griffin CE. Prosthetic heart valves: history of mechanical heart valve replacement. BMES Bulletin 2000; 24: 3–10 passim.

47. Kalke BR, Mantini EL, Morrow AG, Carlson RG, Lillehei CW. Hemodynamic features of a double-leaflet prosthetic heart valve of a new design. Trans Am Soc Artif Intern Organs 1967; 13: 105–110.

48. Starr A, Edwards ML. Mitral replacement: the shielded ball-valve prosthesis. J Thorac Cardiovasc Surg 1961; 42: 673–682.

49. Starr A, Edwards ML. Mitral replacement: clinical experience with a ball-valve prosthesis. Ann Surg 1961; 154: 726–740.

50. Pierie WR, Hancock WD, Koorajian S, Starr A. Materials and heart valve prostheses. Ann NY Acad Sci 1968; 146: 345–359.

51. Lefrak EA, Starr A. Historic aspects of cardiac valve replacement. In Cardiac valve prostheses. New York: Appleton-Century-Crofts, 1979: 3-37.

52. Magovern GJ, Cromie HW. Sutureless prosthetic heart valves. J Thorac Cardiovasc Surg 1963; 46: 726–736.

53. Lefrak EA, Starr A. Magovern–Cromie valve. In Cardiac valve prostheses. New York: Appleton-Century-Crofts, 1979: 129–144.

54. Cartwright RS, Smeloff EA, Davey TB, Kaufman B. Development of a titanium double-caged full-orifice ball valve. Trans Am Soc Artif Intern Organs 1964; 10: 231–236.

55. DeWall RA, Qasim N, Carr L. Evolution of mechanical heart valves. Ann Thorac Surg 2000; 69: 1612–1621.

56. Servelle M, Arbonville G. A ball valve prosthesis with a metallic ball. Surgery 1966; 59: 216–219.

57. Scott SM, Sethi GK, Bridgman AH, Takaro T. Experience with the DeBakey–Surgitool aortic prosthetic valve. Ann Thorac Surg, 1976; 21: 483–486.

58. Leonard F, Nielson CA, Fadali AM, Gott VL. Thromboresistant polymers by emulsion polymerization with anionic surfactants. J Biomed Mater Res 1969; 3: 455–464.

59. Barnard CN, Goosen CC, Holmgren LV, Schrire V. Prosthetic replacement of the mitral valve. Lancet 1962; 2: 1087–1089.

60. Barnard CN, Schrire V, Frater RWM, Goosen CC. Further experiences with the UCT mitral, tricuspid and aortic prostheses. Surgery 1965; 57: 211–219.

61. Melrose DG, Bentall HH, McMillan IKR, Flege JB, Alvarez Diaz FR, Nahas RA, Fautley R, Carson J. The evolution of a mitral-valve prosthesis. Lancet 1964; 2: 623–624.

62. Raftery EB, Dayem MKA, Melrose DG. Mechanical performance of Hammersmith mitral valve prosthesis. Brit Heart J 1968; 30: 666–675.

63. Flege JB, Melrose DG, Bentall HH. Another prosthetic aortic valve: a preliminary report. Ann Thorac Surg 1966; 2: 623–625.

64. Cross FS, Gerein AN, Jone RD. Evaluation of two prosthesis for total replacement of mitral valve. J Thorac Cardiovasc Surg 1963; 46: 719–725.

65. Davila JC. Initial clinical trials of a new, nonthrombogenic mitral-valve prosthesis. Ann Thorac Surg 1968; 6: 99–118.

66. Kay EB. Early years in artificial valve development. Ann Thorac Surg 1989; 48 [Suppl]: S24–S25.

67. Williams KR, Rogers A, Dudrick SJ. Stainless steel disc valve for cardiac valve replacement. J Thorac Cardiovasc Surg 1965; 49: 540–549.

68. Cruz AB, Jr, Kaster RL, Simmons RL, Bruneau L, Lillehei CW. A new caged meniscus prosthetic heart valve. Surgery 1965; 58: 995–998.

69. Kay JH, Kawashima Y, Kagawa Y, Tsuji HK, Redington JV. Experimental mitral valve replacement with a new disc valve. Ann Thorac Surg 1966; 2: 485–498.

70. Kaster RL, Lillehei CW, Helgerud RJ, Rassman WR, Nakib A. The design features and the development of the toroidal prosthetic heart valve. Trans Am Soc Artif Intern Organs 1969; 15: 206–213.

71. Cross FS, Jones RD. A caged-lens prosthesis for replacement of the aortic and mitral valves. Ann Thoracic Surg 1966; 2: 499–505.

72. Beall AC, Bloodwell RD, Liotta D, Cooley DA, DeBakey ME. Clinical experience with a Dacron velour-covered Teflon-disc mitral valve prosthesis. Ann Thorac Surg 1968; 5: 402–410.

73. Harken DE, Matloff JM, Zuckerman W, Chaux A. A new mitral valve. J Thorac Cardiovasc Surg 1968; 55: 369–382.

74. Lefrak EA, Starr A. Starr–Edwards disc valve. In Cardiac valve prostheses. New York: Appleton-Century-Crofts, 1979: 197–204.

75. Lefrak EA, Starr A. Cooley–Cutter valve. In Cardiac valve prostheses. New York: Appleton-Century-Crofts, 1979: 205–214.

76. Barnard PM, Heydenrych JJ, Mead G. Tricuspid valve replacement with the University of Stellenbosch and the University of Cape Town prosthesis: an experimental study. S Afr Med J 1968; 42:250–252.

77. Pierce WS, Behrendt DM, Morrow AG. A hinged prosthetic cardiac valve fabricated of rigid components: experimental evaluations in vitro and in vivo. J Thorac Cardiovasc Surg 1968; 56: 229–235.

78. Wada J, Komatsu S, Ikeda K, Kitaya T, Tanaka N, Yamada H. A new hingeless valve. In Brewer LA III, Ed: Prosthetic heart valves. Springfield: Charles C Thomas, 1989; 304–318.

79. Seidel W, Akutsu T, Mirkovitch V, Kolff WJ. A mitral valve prosthesis and a study of thrombosis on heart valves in dogs. J Surg Res 1962; 2: 168–175.

80. Ernst RW, Stokes HD. An inverted tricuspid plastic mitral valve. J Thorac Cardiovasc Surg 1963; 46: 737–742.

81. Mohri H, Hessel EA, Nelson RJ, Anderson HN, Dillard DH, Merendino KA. Design and durability test of Silastic trileaflet aortic valve prostheses. J Thorac Cardiovasc Surg 1973; 65: 576–582.

82. Timmis HH Discussion in: Frater RWM, Ellis FH Jr. Problems in the development of a mitral valve prosthesis. In Merendino KA, Ed: Prosthetic Valves for Cardiac Surgery. Springfield: Charles C Thomas, 1961; 244–265.

83. Esmond WG, Attar S, Bralley S, McGragor RR, Cowley RA. Design and implantation trials of prosthetic Silastic–Dacron [or Teflon]–Ivalon mitral heart valves. In Merendino KA, Ed: Prosthetic Valves for Cardiac Surgery. Springfield: Charles C Thomas, 1961; 340–367.

84. Schimert G, Sellers RD, Lee CB, Bilgutay AM, Lillehei CW. Fabrication of mitral leaflets and aortic cusps from silastic rubber–coated Teflon felt. In Merendino KA, Ed: Prosthetic Valves for Cardiac Surgery. Springfield:Charles C Thomas, 1961; 368–383.

85. Kay EB, Suzuki A, Postigo J, Nogueira C. Prosthetic replacement of the mitral valve. In Merendino KA, Ed: Prosthetic Valves for Cardiac Surgery. Springfield, Charles C Thomas, 1961; 402–425.

86. Long DM, Gott VL, Sterns LP, Finsterbusch W, Meyne N, Varco RL, Lillehei CW. Reconstruction and replacement of the mitral valve with plastic prostheses. In Merendino KA, Ed: Prosthetic Valves for Cardiac Surgery. Springfield, Charles C Thomas, 1961; 385–401.

87. Muller WH, Littlefield JB, Dammann JF. Subcoronary prosthetic replacement of the aortiv valve. In Merendino KA, Ed: Prosthetic Valves for Cardiac Surgery. Springfield, Charles C Thomas, 1961; 493–507.

88. Malowney RC, Paton BC. A Silastic monocusp mitral prosthesis. J Cardiovasc Surg 1965; 6: 441–446.

89. Duran CG, Gunning AJ. A method for placing a total homologous aortic valve in the subcoronary position. Lancet 1962; 2: 488–489.

90. Ross DN. Homograft replacement of the aortic valve. Lancet 1962; 2: 487–488.

91. Barratt-Boyes BG. Homograft aortic valve replacement in aortic incompetence and stenosis. Thorax 1964; 19: 131–150.

92. Lefrak EA, Starr A. Aortic valve homograft. In Cardiac valve prostheses. New York: Appleton-Century-Crofts, 1979: 273–300.

93. Heimbecker RO, Baird RJ, Lajos TZ, Varga AT, Greenwood WF. Homograft replacement of the human mitral valve. A preliminary report. Can Med Assoc J 1962; 86: 805–809.

94. Angell WW, Wuerflein RD, Shumway NE. Mitral valve replacement with the fresh aortic valve homograft: experimental results and clinical application. Surgery 1967; 62: 807–813.

95. Rogers MA, Chambers RJ, Gotsman MS, Winship WS. Mitral valve replacement with mounted aortic valve homografts. Thorax 1972; 27: 304–310.

96. Lefrak EA, Starr A. Porcine aortic valve xenograft. In: Cardiac valve prostheses. New York: Appleton-Century-Crofts, 1979; 301–329.

97. O'Brien MF, Clarebrough JK. Heterograft aortic valve transplantation for human valve disease. Aust Med J 1966; 2: 228–230.

98. Kaiser GA, Hancock WD, Lukban SB, Litwak RS. Clinical use of a new design stented xenograft heart valve prosthesis. Surg Forum 1969; 20: 137–138.

99. Reis RL, Hancock WD, Yarbrough JW, Glaney DL, Morrow AG. The flexible stent: A new concept in the fabrication of tissue

valve prostheses. J Thorac Cardiovasc Surg 1971; 62: 683–689 passim.

100. Angell WW, Angell JD, Sywak A, Kosek JC. The tissue valve as a superior cardiac valve replacement. Surgery 1977; 82: 875–887.

101. Senning A. Fascia lata replacement of aortic valves. J Thorac Cardiovasc Surg 1967; 54: 465–470.

102. Ionescu MI, Ross DN. Heart-valve replacement with autologous fascia lata. Lancet, 1969; 2: 335–338.

103. Brownlee RT, Yates AK. A fascia lata mitral valve based on the 'frustum' principle. Thorax, 1971; 26: 284–287.

104. McEnany MT, Ross DN, Yates AK. Cusp degeneration in frame-supported autologous fascia lata mitral valves. Thorax, 1972; 27: 23–27.

105. Bodnar E, Bowden NLR, Drury PJ, Olsen EGJ, Durmaz I, Ross DN. Bicuspid mitral bioprosthesis. Thorax, 1981; 36: 45–51.

106. Absolon KB, Hunter SW, Quattlebaum FW. A new technique for cardiac valve construction from autologous diaphragm. Surgery 1959; 46: 1078–1083.

107. Absolon KB. Discussion in: Willman VL, Zafiracopoulos P, Hanlon CR. Replacement of the mitral valve with homograft aortic valve. In Merendino KA, Ed: Prosthetic Valves for Cardiac Surgery. Springfield, Charles C Thomas, 1961; 142–165.

108. Puig LB, Verginelli G, Belotti G, Kawabe L, Frack CCR, Pileggi F, Decourt LV, Zerbini EJ. Homologous dura mater cardiac valve. J Thorac Cardiovasc Surg, 1972; 64: 154–160.

109. Ionescu MI, Pakrashi BC, Holden MP, Mary DAS, Wooler GH. Results from aortic valve replacement with frame supported fascia-lata and pericardial grafts. J Thorac Cardiovasc Surg, 1972; 64: 340–353.

110. Bartek IT, Holden MO, Ionescu MI. Frame-mounted tissue heart valves: technique of construction. Thorax 1974; 29: 51–55.

111. Lefrak EA, Starr A. Bovine pericardial xenograft. In Cardiac valve prostheses. New York: Appleton-Century-Crofts, 1979: 330–340.

112. Vilela Batista RJ, Dobrianskij A, Comazzi M, Lessa Neto LT, Rocha G, Sartori F, Westphal R, Timi JR, Moreira R, Oliveira PF. Clinical experience with stentless pericardial aortic monopatch for aortic valve replacement. J Thorac Cardiovasc Surg 1987; 93: 19–26.

113. Baldwin JT, Campbell A, Luck C, Ogilvie W, Sauter J. Hydrodynamics of the Carbomedics aortic Kinetic prosthetic heart valve. In Piwnica A, Westaby S, Eds: Surgery for acquired aortic valve disease. Oxford: Isis Medical Media 1997; 365–370.

114. Reuters in Health Watch, UK: 17 April 2002.

115. Lefrak EA, Starr A. Björk–Shiley valve. In Cardiac valve prostheses. New York: Appleton-Century-Crofts, 1979: 214–245.

116. Derloshon G. One for the Heart. Irvine: Shiley Incorporated, 1983:89.

117. Björk VO. The central flow tilting disc valve prosthesis (Bjork–Shiley) for mitral valve replacement. Scand J Thorac Cardiovasc Surg 1970; 415–423.

118. Bhuvaneshwar GS, Muraleedharan CV, Vijayan GA, Kumar RS, Valiathan MS. Development of the Chitra tilting disc heart valve prosthesis. J Heart Valve Dis 1996; 5: 448–458.

119. Lillehei CW, Kaster RL, Coleman M, Bloch JH. Heart-valve replacement with Lillehei–Kaster pivoting disc prosthesis. NY State Med J 1974; 74: 1426–1438.

120. Starek PJ, McLaurin LP, Wilcox BR, Murray GF. Clinical evaluation of the Lillehei–Kaster pivoting-disc valve. Ann Thorac Surg 1976; 22: 362–368.

121. Hall KV. The Medtronic Hall heart valve. Background, latest results, and future work. Ann Thorac Surg 1989; 48 [Suppl]: S47–S48.

122. Reul H, Steinseifer U, Knoch M, Rau G. Development, manufacturing and validation of single leaflet mechanical heart valve prosthesis. J Heart Valve Dis 1995; 4: 513–519.

123. Barton K, Campbell A, Chinn JA, Griffin CD, Hern-Anderson D, Klein K, Moore MA, Zapanta C. Prosthetic heart valves: current and future perspectives. BMES Bulletin 2001; 25: 3–16 passim.

124. Myers D. New tissue processing techniques. In Piwnica A, Westaby S, Eds: Surgery for acquired aortic valve disease. Oxford: Isis Medical Media 1997; 448-456.

125. Lefrak EA, Starr A. Bovine pericardial xenograft. In Cardiac valve prostheses. New York: Appleton-Century-Crofts, 1979: 330–340.

126. Rosen JJ, Wright JT, Myers DJ, Johansen J. Hydrodynamic performance of a new pericardial heart valve.Trans Am Soc Artif Intern Organs 1981; 27: 151–154.

127. Gabbay S, Bortolotti U, Cipolletti G, Wasserman F, Frater RW, Factor SM. The Meadox unicusp pericardial bioprosthetic heart valve: new concept. Ann Thorac Surg 1984; 37: 448–456.

128. Neethling WM, Papadimitriou JM, Swarts E, Hodge AJ. Kangaroo versus porcine aortic valve tissue-valve geometry morphology, tensile strength and calcification potential. J Cardiovasc Surg [Torino] 2000; 41: 341–348.

129. Murakami T. Experimental studies of original valved conduit using glutaraldehyde-preserved equine pericardium (Xenomedica). Hokkaido Igaku Zasshi 1989; 64: 286–300.

130. Angell WW, Grehl TM, Buch W, Waerflein RD. Mounted fresh homograftfor aortic valve replacement. Med J Aust 1972; 2 [Suppl]: 74–76.

131. Heng MK, Barratt–Boyes B, Agnew TM, Brandt PW, Kerr AR, Graham KJ. Isolated mitral replacement with stent-mounted antibiotic-treated aortic allograft valves. J Thorac Cardiovasc Surg 1977; 74: 230–237.

132. Chaukar AP, Patwardhan AM, Kaul A, Borker SS. Homograft valve revisited. Indian J Thorac Cardiovasc Surg 1993; 9: 78–80.

133. Bhattacharya S, Vinchurkar M, Kaul A, Patwardhan AM, Chaukar AP. Stent design and in vitro studies of homograft bioprostheses. Indian J Thorac Cardiovasc Surg 1993; 9: 81–85.

134. David TE, Ropchan GC, Butany JW. Aortic valve replacement with stentless porcine bioprostheses. J Cardiac Surg 1988; 3: 501–505.

135. Levy D, Garrison RJ, Savage DD, Kannel WB, Castelli WP. Prognostic implications of echocardiographically determined left ventricular mass in the Framingham Heart Study. N Engl J Med 1990; 322: 1561–1566.

136. Lund O. Valve replacement for aortic stenosis: the curative potential of early operation. Scand J Thor Cardiovasc Surg 1993; 40 [Suppl]: 1–137.

137. Frater RWM, Liao K, Seifter E. Stentless chordally supported mitral bioprosthetic valve. New Horizon 1994; 103–119.

138. Walther T, Walther C, Falk V, Diegeler A, Krakor R, Schneider J, Autschbach R, Mohr FW. Early clinical results after stentless mitral valve implantation and comparison with conventional valve repair or replacement. Circulation 1999; 100 [Suppl]: II-78–II-83.

139. Westaby S, Bianco RW, Katsumata T, Termin P. Semin Thorac Cardiovasc Surg 1999; 11[Suppl]: 206–209.

140. Park SZ, Reardon MJ. Current status of stentless aortic xenografts. Curr Opin Cardiol, 2000; 15: 74–81.

141. O'Brien MF, Goldstein S, Walsh S, Black KS, Elkins R, Clarke D. The SynerGraft valve: A new acellular (nonglutaraldehyde-fixed) tissue heart valve for autologous recellularization. First experimental studies before clinical implantation. Semin Thorac Cardiovasc Surg 1999;11 [Suppl]: 194–200.

142. Sievers HH, Stierle U, Schmidtke C, Bechtel M. Decellularized pulmonary homograft (SynerGraft) for reconstruction of the right ventricular outflow tract. First clinical experience. Z Kardiol 2003; 92: 53–59.

143. Sodian R, Hoerstrup SP, Sperling JS, Daebritz S, Martin DP, Moran AM, Kim BS, Schoen FJ, Vacanti JP, Mayer JE Jr. Early in vivo experience with tissue-engineered trileaflet heart valves. Circulation 2000; 102 [Suppl]: III 22–III 29.

144. Irwin E, Lang G, Clack R, St Cyr J, Runge W, Foker J, Bianco R. Long term evaluation of prosthetic mitral valves in sheep. J Invest Surg 1993; 6:133–141.

145. Davies H. Catheter–mounted valve for temporary relief of aortic insufficiency. Lancet, 1965; 1: 250.

146. Moulopoulos SD, Anthopoulos L, Stametelopoulos S, Stefadouros M. Catheter–mounted aortic valves. Ann Thorac Surg 1971; 11: 423–430.

147. Andersen HR, Knudsen LL, Hasenkam JM. Transluminal implantation of artificial heart valves. Description of a new expandable aortic valve and initial results with implantation by catheter technique in closed chest pigs. Eur Heart J 1992; 13: 704–708.

148. Bonhoeffer P, Boudjemline Y, Saliba Z, Hausse AO, Aggoun Y, Bonnet D, Sidi D, Kachaner J. Transcatheter implantation of a bovine valve in pulmonary position: a lamb study. Circulation 2000; 102: 813–816.

149. Bonhoeffer P, Boudjemline Y, Saliba Z, Merckx J, Aggoun Y, Bonnet D, Acar P, Le Bidois J, Sidi D, Kachaner J. Percutaneous replacement of pulmonary valve in a right-ventricle to pulmonary-artery prosthetic conduit with valve dysfunction. Lancet 2000; 356[9239]:1403–1405.

150. Boudjemline Y, Bonhoeffer P. Steps toward percutaneous aortic valve replacement. Circulation 2002; 105: 775–778.

151. Cribier A, Eltchaninoff H, Bash A, Borenstein N, Tron C, Bauer F, Derumeaux G, Anselme F, Laborde F, Leon MB. Percutaneous transcatheter implantation of an aortic valve prosthesis for calcific aortic stenosis: first human case description. Circulation 2002; 106: 3006–3008.

152. Banerjee A, Mathew SG. Blueprint for a quadrileaflet arotic valve prosthesis. Indian Heart J 2000; 52: 615–617.

Permission

The illustrations listed below have been reprinted with the permission of their respective copyright-owners/ publishers, as indicated:

Figure No	Permission–granting authority	Ref No
003	Elsevier Science/ American Association for Thoracic Surgery	3
004	American College of Surgeons	4
005,009	Westminster Publications /Angiology Research Foundation	5
007	American College of Surgeons	80
08	Elsevier Science/ The Society of Thoracic Surgeons	11
013	Elsevier Science/ The Society of Thoracic Surgeons	16
015,016,017	Elsevier Science/ American Association for Thoracic Surgery	17
018	Lippincott, Williams and Wilkins	18
019	Elsevier Science/ American Association for Thoracic Surgery	19
020	South African Medical Association	21
022	Elsevier Science/ American Association for Thoracic Surgery	24
023	Elsevier Science/ American Association for Thoracic Surgery	25
024,025	Mayo Clinic Proceedings	26
030	The American Physiological Society	32
031	John Wiley and Sons Ltd/ British Journal of Surgery Society Ltd	34
032,033	South African Medical Association	35
036	Texas Heart institute Journal	43
045,046,049,050	Appleton–Century–Crofts	51

067,068	Elsevier Science/ The Lancet	61
071	Elsevier Science/ The Society of Thoracic Surgeons	63
072	Elsevier Science/ American Association for Thoracic Surgery	64
078	Elsevier Science/ American Association for Thoracic Surgery	67
085	Elsevier Science/ The Society of Thoracic Surgeons	71
086	Elsevier Science/ The Society of Thoracic Surgeons	72
098	Elsevier Science/ Academic Press	79
100	Elsevier Science/ American Association for Thoracic Surgery	81
119	BMJ Publishing Group	95
121,129	Elsevier Science/ American Association for Thoracic Surgery	99
124	Elsevier Science/ The Lancet	102
125	BMJ Publishing Group	103
127	Elsevier Science/ American Association for Thoracic Surgery	108
130	Elsevier Science/ American Association for Thoracic Surgery	112
202	American society of Artificial Internal Organs	126
203	Elsevier Science/ The Society of Thoracic Surgeons	127
268	Elsevier Science/ American Association for Thoracic Surgery	141
275	Elsevier Science/ The Lancet	145

www.heartcenteronline.com
www.heartlab.rri.on.ca
www.heartpoint.com
www.heartvalves.com
www.hsforum.com
www.ibb.gatech.edu
www.icr-heart.com
www.imrser.org
www.invibio.com
www.jyros.com
www.lerner.ccf.org
www.lpch.org
www.mcritx.com
www.med.umich.edu
www.medal.org
www.medcvinc.com
www.medtronic.com
www.mgh.harvard.edu
www.mitroflow.com
www.netdoctor.co.uk
www.nlm.nih.gov
www.onevalveforlife.com
www.openheartsurgery.com
www.perimount.com.
www.rds-online.org.uk
www.shvd.org
www.sjm.com
www.sorin-cid.com
www.stanfordhospital.com
www.st-jude-heart-valve.com
www.stjudemedical.com
www.sts.org
www.texheartsurgeons.com
www.tmc.edu
www.washington.edu
www.3ftherapeutics.com
heart.uchospitals.edu
heart-surgeon.com
info.med.yale.edu
members.evansville.net

- Mr S Khalid Husain, Mr Nishat Alam and the staff of Express Colour Scan; Dr Bandana Malhotra, Dr Ratnamalika Kumar and Ms Anjana Bhatia for their assistance in preparation of the manuscript.
- Mr Sanu Kapila, Mr Rituraj Kapila and the staff of Academic Foundation; and Mr Shobit Arya of Print Perfect for executing the finale of this book.

Dr Amit Banerjee is professor of cardiovascular–thoracic surgery at the Govind Ballabh Pant Hospital, New Delhi, a postdoctoral training institution devoted to higher medical specialities. It is affiliated to Delhi University and associated with the Maulana Azad Medical College—rated as one of the best medical colleges in India. Born in 1949, he completed his graduate and postgraduate medical education from this college. He qualified as a cardiothoracic surgeon in 1980 from the institution he serves today.

Dr Banerjee's areas of special interest include surgical treatment for atrial fibrillation associated with valvular heart disease and noncoronary open heart operations on beating heart. He is a former editor of the *Indian Journal of Thoracic and Cardiovascular Surgery.*

Delving into the history of cardiac surgery, especially the evolution of equipment, instruments and devices, constitutes Dr Banerjee's favourite pastime. He is also a keen student of medical philately. He was instrumental in conceptualising perhaps the one and only postage stamp, along with a first–day cover and a special postal cancellation (pictured below), commemorating the Centenary of Cardiac Surgery, released by His Excellency the President of India in 1996.

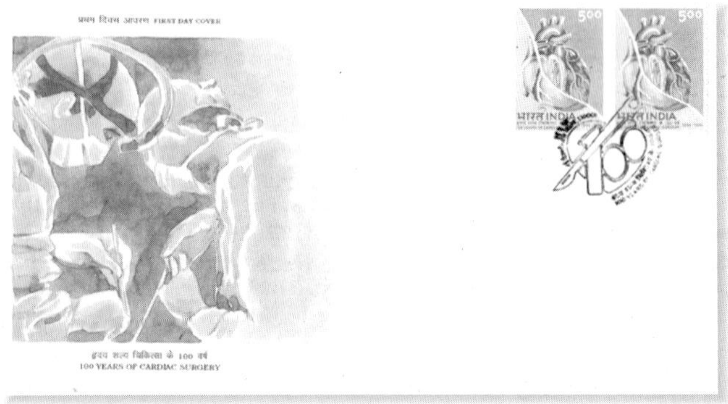